Hargrave Jennings

Phallicism

celestial and terrestrial, heathen and Christian, its connexion with the Rosicrucians

and the Gnostics and its foundation in Buddhism, with an essay on mystic anatomy

Hargrave Jennings

Phallicism
celestial and terrestrial, heathen and Christian, its connexion with the Rosicrucians and the Gnostics and its foundation in Buddhism, with an essay on mystic anatomy

ISBN/EAN: 9783337246853

Printed in Europe, USA, Canada, Australia, Japan

Cover: Foto ©Andreas Hilbeck / pixelio.de

More available books at **www.hansebooks.com**

PHALLICISM

CELESTIAL AND TERRESTRIAL

HEATHEN AND CHRISTIAN

ITS CONNEXION WITH THE ROSICRUCIANS AND THE GNOSTICS AND ITS FOUNDATION IN BUDDHISM

WITH AN ESSAY ON MYSTIC ANATOMY

BY

HARGRAVE JENNINGS

AUTHOR OF "THE ROSICRUCIANS," ETC. ETC.

LONDON

GEORGE REDWAY

YORK STREET COVENT GARDEN

MDCCCLXXXIV.

CONTENTS.

viii

Contents.

Notice.—A small series of engravings illustrative of the subject of the present work is in preparation, under the superintendence of a gentleman connected with the British Museum, and will be issued, with letterpress descriptions, in a convenient form, for presentation to subscribers.

Those who may care for this supplement will please notify their wishes to the publisher, in order that a copy may be forwarded, for which there is no charge whatever; but in no case will the illustrations be supplied through agents, or otherwise than on direct application to THE PUBLISHER.

INTRODUCTION.

ALL these original facts and theories, as applicable to general religion, were first brought forward by the author in a work entitled, "The Indian Religions; or, Results of the Mysterious Buddhism," published in the early part of the year 1858. Subsequently to the appearance of that book several other writers, impressed by its importance, hitherto unsuspected, took up and enlarged upon the details referring to this subject, without, however, touching, or seeming to be even aware of, the spirit and inner meaning of the matters which they so confidently and ignorantly handled, with, however, all the innocent good faith in the world. This exploration into the modern day refers to the recurrence of the introduction into history of the "PHALLIC THEORY," as supplying the necessarily mystic groundwork of ALL RELIGION— nay, furnishing altogether the reasons *for* religion. Conspicuous among these writers, subsequent in time to the production of the work above referred to, is Dr. Thomas Inman, of Liverpool, a writer of singular ingenuity, but astray in his general disbelieving conclusions, his particulars being correct, while his results are arrived at erroneously, though in full sincerity, which is deeply to be regretted, considering the display of so much indefatigable research and the expenditure of so much valuable labour. Dr. Inman is the author of two ponderous, very learned volumes, entitled, "ANCIENT FAITHS

b

EMBODIED IN ANCIENT NAMES." To a certain extent there is a similarity in this valuable work to that of Godfrey Higgins, which displayed wonderful penetration and power of analysis, and indomitable philosophical insight, enthusiasm, hardihood and perseverance, published under the title of "ANACALYPSIS; OR, AN ATTEMPT TO DRAW ASIDE THE VEIL OF THE SAITIC ISIS," in heavy quarto volumes, in 1833, 1834, 1836. The "CELTIC DRUIDS," another important quarto of Godfrey Higgins, abounding in antiquarian truth, and beautifully illustrated, appeared in 1829; and, in 1834, an invaluable antiquarian Phallic book, "THE ROUND TOWERS OF IRELAND," written by a very accomplished scholar, Henry O'Brien, who, of course, mainly on account of his insight, solidity, and genuineness, especially as advocating—nay, proving—unwelcome and startling antiquarian conclusions in regard to the ROUND TOWERS, encountered not much less than a storm of opposition. These books (we may aver), on account of their difficult, evading and reluctant (even obstinate) subjects for discovery, range under the same head as Dr. Inman's "ANCIENT FAITHS." They explain idolatry.

Messrs. Staniland Wake and Westropp, and Dr. Phené, a well-known and industrious antiquary, produced memoranda and books of greater or less importance and noteworthiness upon this strange but engrossingly seductive "Phallic" subject, when their attention had been led up to it;—though, in truth, the emulative attention of these scholars was first challenged by the works in which the topic was dilated upon (but only in the certain proper way) by the present writer.

The curiosity in regard to this subject spread, as was

to be expected. Efforts at the disinterment of the conclusions of the ancient mystical writers, taken up from point to point, followed on the writings of the present author. The Americans in particular, in circuitous deflections or more promising direct searching out, wrote and published in recognitive quarters. And this movement evoked sparks of re-animation to the truths of the Phallic theory in various directions back again in our own country. Through these means was incited notice to these grand philosophical problems of the real meaning of the old idolatries in which lay the expression of enthusiastic religion. The seeds, cast at hazard originally with much distrust of their reception in this present too-sharpened intellectual age, took root in the New World. The mainly forgotten puzzles among our inquisitive brethren in America found fit matrix in which to spring. And in response to this antiquarian signal, sounded across the seas, books in America made their appearance, arising principally from certain abstract (and before that time unconsidered, except by Sir William Jones, the great Indian authority,) speculations as to the groundwork of that shadowy religion—" mystery of all mysteries"—Buddhism—handled nowadays by very many and very incompetent hands. These original ideas about Buddhism were published by the present writer in his work "The Indian Religions," which contains the germ of all the new views. But all these discourses by other people, and speculative attempts to discover—this hovering for ever round and round a subject, more than general description of which is denied, and which is ever intended to be denied—even in the mental interest of the querists themselves—have been vain, because they have been insufficient, formed out of that which could sustain no structure, and springing from minds not abstract and keen enough to find out for themselves—being not adequately gifted.

There is always a fixed point of reserve in these occult matters, beyond which it is hopeless—as it has always been, and always must be—to penetrate. Large and important enough is the margin up to this rigid line, beyond which, to all ordinary explorers, access and dis-covery is as impossible as it would be uncomfortable, if by any possibility of comprehension arrival at these grand supernatural truths could ever be realised—that is, by the usual inost acute inquirers among the people. But the majority of investigators—even learned investigators—are dull enough, and are too cold of imagination to be im-pressed with great facts if they happen to be remote ideas and new and difficult to be believed. Therefore all is at the best in this general incredibility. And the secrets are so fixed and so sure—being so deep-buried for all time in symbols so mysterious as to be far beyond reading—that the paraded decipherments, to those knowing ones whose attention has been drawn to them through the aggressive vanity of the Egyptologists and in the effrontery of some of the predominating scientific people, although trumpeted in the Press as discoveries, are laughed at quietly by those who " know better." But the persuading of the public is easy by the strength of names, and through the." influence of authority in matters of opinion,"—a persuasion which did not escape the penetration of Sir George Cornewall Lewis, nor does it evade the detection of certain cool observers disposed to pass over with a certain measure of contempt the parade of the string of letters—marking degrees—which, like the paper vertebræ of the flexile tail of a kite—adorn many a name stamped with the stamps of academical and other supposed and accepted learned societies.

The present writer furthermore claims to be the first introducer, as the grand philosophical problem, of the vast religious and national importance of "Buddhism," so important to England, as being the mistress of India, of the immense Buddhistic countries, with their prodigious populations. Buddhism and its speculative foundations, and the question whether these are founded in absolute vital truth, or whether they are to be dismissed as mere mythology, has now become such an important topic that no words can realise the extent and possible results of the same.

The attestation to the justice of his claim is to be found in the fact of the number of books upon the subject of Buddhism which have appeared since the date of the "Indian Religions; or, Results of the Mysterious Buddhism," produced in the years of the great Indian Mutiny—viz., 1857-1858. This book — a moderate-sized octavo — although entirely opposed to the arguments and line of indoctrination of nearly the whole of the British Press and the political people, headed by the *Times,* and to the opinions enunciated and approved by the general ratification of the people of England (in appearance), was warmly adopted and certified as establishing truths by no less distinguished and enthusiastic and patriotic authorities than a previous Governor-General, the Earl of Ellenborough; by Sir Erskine Perry, Judge of the Supreme Court of Bombay, and several other members of the

Council of India; by Lord Lyndhurst, the Lord Chancellor, many members of Parliament, principally from the Conservative ranks, and many scholars and enlightened men, not only in France and England, but in Germany, and particularly in the United States of America, where these subjects were viewed largely, apart from politics. We may declare that the book was received with great marks of favour—this, in its explanations, as speaking truth (and useful, enlightening truth), in regard to the real opinions and feelings of the vast population of India, both of the Hindoos and the Mahometans. Notwithstanding this, it was truth, necessarily unpopular and disbelieved in at that time—now long past—provoking and enraging in the then natural fierceness of feeling and in the impulse of intense hostility in England to everything (native) of India. This work, "The Indian Religions," now totally out of print and very scarce, was published anonymously, and was founded upon a mass of authoritative proofs furnished to the author from India itself. It bore—at once an entreaty and a warning— upon its title-page the significant words of Themistocles in his own native Greek, as applied and addressed to the people of England, "Strike, but hear!"

It was really a very bold challenge offered to public opinion in England—so aroused, and so, as the present writer thought at the time, mistaken—this laying before the people of England such a remonstrance in regard to the general unfortunate policy. Of the mistakes of this policy the British people are now thoroughly convinced.

In some very eminent but at that time unpopular quarters in England (1857-1858) this novel and unexpected anonymous work secured deep attention and won firm reliance. But although too bitterly true, as the book called in question the entire round of opinion and of decision, in regard to remedies, as pronounced in England through the Press, and as emanating from the authorities, and confirmed and authorised by Parliament (then aroused to the intensest spirit of indignation and of excitement), its arguments were considered as incredible, and its statements as too extraordinary, and as too truly unexpected, when announced as coming from (of all people in the world) an "Indian Missionary," as was stated on the title-page. This authorship and this origin were very naturally regarded as a phenomenon when the "Indian Missionary" appeared as the apologist on the Indian side. He was only arguing, however, for truth. He offered real evidence. The judicious people, on consideration, discovered, to the general amazement, that the foundations of Buddhism had been hitherto wholly misunderstood. It was realised at last that these foundations were not only mystical and unexplainable—because occult and cabalistic—not only impossible of denial, (that is, in their "results" or conclusions)—but that they were true. The difficulty, especially in this country, is to make new ideas, and new and apparently contradictory views of things, understood, above all (and inveterately so) in the case of religion. There is an amount of prejudice inconceivable to all who have not been either compelled or have elected to move in the face of it.

("Have you not heard," says Mr. William Morris, "how it has gone with many a cause before now? First, few men heed it. Next, most men contemn it. Lastly, all men accept it. And the cause is won!")

Mr. Gerald Massey, in his "Natural Genesis and Typology of Primitive Customs," has drawn his ideas upon very important mythic subjects from a remote source. Comparatively speaking, he has thus ´rendered them second-hand. He has gained his notions from the "Indian Religions; or, The Results of the Mysterious Buddhism," and the "Curious Things of the Outside World," respectively published so long ago, and more particularly from the "Rosicrucians," in its first edition, published early in 1870.

Truly, in certain respects, Mr. Gerald Massey has read wrongly, and has been over-eager. He has traced erroneously the outlining of his conceptions when his originals seemed somewhat restive in his own mistaking hands. Mr. Gerald Massey's two ponderous tomes, "The Book of the Beginnings," present, in the first instance, the very serious fault of being greatly too bulky, and the book is far too expensive for general acceptance and circulation. In addition, the work is uninviting from its diffusiveness, and it labours under the singular demerit that, whilst many of its particulars are correct, and its groups of facts to a large extent trustworthy, the general deductions therefrom are wholly mistaken. They are guide-posts which indicate to those who consult and spell them over, in curiosity and hope, the wrong paths. It is certainly most inauspicious in the interests of the profounder students of these difficult subjects that this unintended although bewildering maze of erroneous results from apparently correct particulars should be so confidently paraded. For doubt and continual distrust are the parents of successful discovery.

As if all the mysteries—reluctant enough to previous

inquirers—had miraculously opened out of themselves to the new examiner, and had satisfactorily disclosed themselves to the discovery of one man in the latter time! Such overweening confidence is most absurd and most disastrous. Truly must we be forced to consider that all previous great men and the long line of profound thinkers —labouring through the ages—had worked in vain. Mr. Gerald Massey's text is that all religions and all mysteries evolved from out of the heart of Africa. We simply reject all his accumulation of particulars as founded on a wrong basis. The effect of such books is only to clog the subject and to confuse the reader.

We prefer other claims to the reader's consideration. The present book may be undoubtedly pronounced new and perfectly original. It is professedly constructive. It finds its justification in an elaborate consideration of the monuments of the old world, and in the usages and ideas of the moderns. It is most important in one respect. It seeks to be the builder up of a belief—of a CHRISTIAN belief. This, in opposition to most modern books of its nature. It will be found strange, puzzling, startling. But all its conclusions will be supported by abundant proofs—to the right-minded and to the most accomplished and the most deeply-read among the antiquaries.

Curious and inquisitive readers will find in it all that they want to know concerning that extremely recondite and interesting subject. The Phallic ideas will be discovered herein, upon indisputable evidence, to be the foundation of ALL RELIGIONS. The tokens and traces of this peculiar—and, as it became in its treatment by the peoples of antiquity, this refined and picturesque— worship are to be recognised as deeply sunk in the

art and architecture of all nations. Phallicism gave
richness, colour, and poetical variety to all the myths.
Furthermore, these indications are detected as lying
purposely and felicitously concealed (but only in their
own pure method of acceptation) in all the insignia of the
Christian Church. This at every point where mysterious-
ness (and therefore truth) commences, and where plain-
teaching (or the practical) ceases. It may be very safely
assumed as a distinguishing fact in the examination of the
work that just in proportion to the knowledge, learning,
and taste of the reader will be the quickness of his
discovery, recognition, and appreciation.

It is really believed that almost every book, in whatever
language, from which anything of import could be
obtained towards the flood of light (within the proper
bounds) cast upon this fascinating subject, has been
examined and adduced in evidence. The mystic sexual
anatomy, as bearing upon religion, and the "whys" and
the "wherefores" of the necessarily occult existence
of these curious subjects, have been carefully gone
into.

The work will assume, as a sort of ground truth, that
this contemporaneous—greatly too self-sufficient and too
self-reliant—time remains too complacently confident in
its own conclusions. The present age has made up its
mind as to that which is to be believed and that which is
not to be believed. There is certainly no want of books
to enter largely into an examination of the religious ideas
and systems which have prevailed in all ages. Religion
of some sort, and an acknowledgment of the gods, is
necessary for man. Histories—more or less able, and
books informing people, in the greater or lesser degree,

of that which they did not know before—are continually
appearing. Memoirs, theses, and accounts, orthodox,
critical, and explanatory, some with much learning and
indicative of considerable labour, trace out the original
footsteps of the nations, which, according to the earliest
notions connected with the progress of the human race,
set out, seeking new places of settlement and more
convenient and inviting homes. But, like most of those
who have descried first—and then traced—the reappear-
ance of Indian religions, ideas, and myths in Egypt, in
Persia, in Europe, in the most remote directions even in
America—querists—truly the most undaunted and resolute querists—have thought that they ended when they
pointed out the similarity.

Those who are surprised to find the tenacity of these
Phallic vestiges, and that they are all to be re-read in
the Egyptian and in the Greek and Roman systems of
theological construction, and in their monuments, seem to
think that the wonder disappears, and that the riddle has
been read, when these strange things are seen reduced
into order and are evident in their new home. On the
contrary, the fact is that the wonder, instead of being
explained, is only just beginning. The problem, instead
of being resolved, has only just shifted its place, and is
as much a problem still.

All religions commence in myths and disappear in
myths ;—because the ends and purposes of life—of man
altogether—the meaning of nature itself—are wrapped
up in mystery. In the present work the author's object
is to show that the modern time owes everything to
the ancient. There is not a form, an idea, a grace,
a sentiment, a felicity in art which is not owing, in

one form or another, to the Phallicism, and its' means of indication, which at one time in the monuments—statuesque, architectural—covered the whole earth. All this has been ignored—averted from—carefully concealed (together with all the philosophy which went with it), because it has been judged indecent. As if anything seriously resting in nature, and being notoriously everything in nature and art (everything at least that is grand and beautiful), could be—apart from the mind making it so—indecent.

It may be at once boldly asserted as a truth that there is not a religion that does not spring from the sexual distinctions. All these great facts have been obliterated. In the present work an attempt has been made to do justice to the greatness and majesty of the ancients, and to exhibit their ideas of religion, and of the character of religion, as true—though necessarily clouded over (or rather illustrated) with allegory (mythologies), as the truths of all religions must be—naked truth never being intended for man.

Thus we are pre-eminently constructive. The work will be found to contain a complete survey of the rationale of Buddhism and its philosophical inflections and the depths of its mystic ideas. In regard to Buddhism and to its purpose and foundation—whether true or false—the world is in a state of greater contention than ever at the present period. This is witnessed by the numerous books which continually appear, treating of Buddhism and of the theories concerning it. It will be found that, reposing upon the abstractions of Buddhism, the network of mythological allegory which has been raised over it, and the mystic dogmas which have been embraced in it, have refined, and metamorphosed, and spread, and fitted, and adapted themselves into the beliefs of other countries, the widest separated in time and place.

It is a noteworthy fact—a guiding principle in the influences of civilisation all over the world—that all religions and all forms of religion—preternatural, as we contend, and enlightened in man's receptivity (or soul), from the original design and intention of a PERSONAL PROVIDENCE—have started from the centre of Asia. The arts of life and the systems of living in community— the gradual coalescing and amalgamation and the settle- ment of nations—have moved majestically in the sublime march of the centuries—"tiring out Time," as it really seems to us—contemplating, in these latter days (when a general impatience seems to beset all mankind); these latter days, full of evil, full of fear, self-conceit, weariness, confusion, and woe, from the East, all round the world, to the West. The mind of man has moved forth from the Tigris and the Euphrates—only become errant when "*driven out*"—out from the allegorical "Garden;" in after time from Balkh (with foundation unknown), the Mother and Anarch of Cities, or as the commencement of a previous new era to the world, or to a new dispen- sation, from the Mountain of the Ark, or the Cradle of Humanity, following the course of the latitudes West- ward and tracking the Sun to the Westernmost shores of the New World. Here, arrested by the mighty Pacific Ocean, which seems the grand barrier to mankind and his designs—"Thus far shalt thou come, but no farther" —along that never-ending line, ranging athwart the world, the histories of man seem to culminate. Perhaps here, on the shore of the far—the *farthest*—West, where the

" tired civilisations" seem rousing up as for a new display
—having made the whole circle of the earth—the rest-
less demonstrative communities, with their inventions and
astonishments (how unlike the tranquil greatness of the
ancients!) may subside to peace.   For a second new
promenade of the peoples of the world around the earth
seems unlikely.

Enormous labour—the labour of many years—and an
enthusiasm which was converted out of the utmost original
disbelief of these wondrously stimulating and beautiful
Phallic beliefs;—all this curious inquest into the meaning
and reality of the Phallicism which lies at the root of all
religions—as also of the Christian religion—pains, trouble,
and suspicious examination until convinced, have gone to
the compilation of the present book.   Its chief merit, or
at least one of its choice merits, is its conciseness and
brevity.   It comprises, within the limits of a modest
octavo, all that can be known (or, at least, all that is
permitted to be known by prudent, competent persons)
of the doctrines of the BUDDHISTS, GNOSTICS, and
ROSICRUCIANS, as connected with " Phallicism."

We have gone over the whole ground with care to
distinguish.   We have filled up with details of the primitive worship of the creative principle, under such symbols
as the Obelisk, Pillar, and Pyramid.   We have traced
the division of sects, and have discriminated in the character of the Phallic monuments, whether as referring to
the preference of the Lunar influence or of the Solar power,
as the cause of the earliest wars and of the " primæval
dispersion."   An endeavour has been made to effect this
history of the monuments of antiquity, not in the spirit
and in the manner of the antiquary and compiler only,

but with the object of the recovery of a faith, believing (as we do) that the peoples of antiquity had excellent reasons for what they did, and were actuated by a fine and true instinct. It will very readily be perceived that the element of faith is necessary to the proper apprehension of the reality and seriousness of the array of real matters which we pass in review. Nothing strikes forcibly, or arrests the attention efficaciously, which is not believed in by the writer, and the absence of this reliance is very soon detected.

Not to burthen our pages with small type and interrupt the narrative with subsidiary, confirmatory matter in the places where it is not so readily to be looked for, we have decided to relegate to an Appendix certain notes of value in elucidation, and transcripts of facts and items of evidence. These will be found to materially help the reader to a proper and consecutive understanding of the subject.

A subject lying so out of sight in the ordinarily beaten historical paths—in regard of which we have truly so much investigation and such exposition so reiterated that it wearies—will of course be found abstruse and difficult to reconcile with ordinary conclusions to those whose attention before this has not been called thereto and to those who have not hitherto made it a special study.

The various accounts, and the conjectures more or less happily hazarded, given by different authors respecting the reality and meaning—philosophically and vitally—of the Phallic worship, and why its prevalence should have been so great in olden times, will not a little serve to puzzle the reader and to upset the foregone conclusions which he has derived in the course of his education.

He will find, indeed, that he has much to be enlightened concerning, if he has not diligently sought for knowledge at the right sources, for the proper understanding of these religious aberrations, and to comprehend the deep impression which the unseen world (to the shame of the moderns) held over the ancients.

In this book will be found a more complete and more connected account than has hitherto appeared of the different forms of the worship (which has distinguished all ages), or peculiar veneration (not idolatry), generally denominated the Phallic worship. No previous writer has disserted so fully upon the shades and varieties of this singular ritual, or traced up so completely its mysterious blendings with the ideas of the philosophers, as to what lies remotely in Nature in regard to the origin and history of the human race. The well-known work of Richard Payne Knight is a mine of learned matter bearing upon this subject; but it is devoted more especially to the rites which celebrated the worship of Priapus among the Romans.

The antiquarian world has yet to do justice to the memory of Henry O'Brien, a most penetrating antiquary, who—gifted particularly and richly by nature—soon perceived the folly and inconsequence of the conclusions afloat in his day in regard to the Round Towers of Ireland. Among the competition essays as to the origin and destination of these famous Round Towers, furnished in answer to the desire to settle this point, if possible, by the offer of its first prize or gold medal, by the Royal Irish Academy, in 1833—34, appeared one essay— which proved to be by O'Brien—that should properly have settled the debate for ever. Its arguments and proofs, in justice to its well-directed learning, should have been accepted at once. However—as is generally the case in these remote and difficult inquiries—O'Brien was disbelieved. Owing to the want of resolute and quick-sighted capacity to judge accurately, the usual pur-blind conclusion was arrived at. Notwithstanding this conspicuous failure of literary justice the striking merits of O'Brien's masterly treatise made themselves evident in a certain degree, and the *second* prize was adjudged to this piece, while the gold medal and the first place were assigned to an essay by Dr. Petrie—another Irish antiquary—whose notions, being commonplace, were safegoing and plausible, and better agreed with the temper of the adjudicators. Dr. Petrie refused to allow of the extreme antiquity of the Round Towers, gave them a Christian origin, and assigned to their erection a much later date. Never was incompetence made more manifest. Poor Henry O'Brien died a young man, having, when in London, become one of the chief contributors, in his own particular line of antiquities, to *Fraser's Magazine* at the time of its highest distinc-tion. He wrote and laboured with all the en-thusiasm of a cultured Irishman, and with the correctness of a sage. His book upon the " Round Towers" is now acknowledged as the only correct book, and the *best* book, upon the subject. It has become very scarce, and is eagerly bought up wherever encountered.

Edward Sellon—to whose care, knowledge, and dis-crimination the world is indebted for the arrangement of the choice Phallic collection in the British Museum—has furnished an account of the Phallic worship in India only, which is authenticated by passages in the writings of

Sir William Jones, Wilford, and other historians, travellers, and commentators, more or less skilled and prepared
by study.

The most painstaking and indefatigable of all these
explorers into the foundations of the old religions is
Godfrey Higgins. But he loses sight of the great contention implied in the very cause in wading amidst
the labyrinths of evidence. The question in reality is
not whether the forms of the religion are true, but
whether religion itself is true. We believe that it
is, and we have written accordingly—that is, to CON-
STRUCT. Godfrey Higgins has given to the world—like
Thomas Inman and others—marvellous books, monuments of industry and of expense. But they reduce
religion to a mechanical exercise. They are historical
accounts of rites, ceremonies, and usages—and how they
have passed in the practice of all the peoples—matters,
truths, and relations which nobody disputes. The machinery of a religion, or of all religion, every person can
understand. That which impels the machinery is the
great subject to be discussed.

To explain the symbols and the mysticism always
accompanying them, together with the recondite references to the unsuspected powers of Nature implied in
the imagery—often a purposed dream or " masquerade"
—of the celebrated Gnostic gems ;—to decipher the
hieroglyphics which puzzle strangers to these curious
subjects ;—to elucidate the meanings conveyed in the
monuments and relics, sculpturesque and architectural—
all expressive of something of moment to be transmitted
and communicated,—left as a legacy, as it were, by the
old times to the later times,—all this, which, of course,

is the aim of all writers, is a work of difficulty, which must be still further aggravated unless the reader is surrounded by books of prints, or by the actual gems, statues, sculpture, to which reference in the text is made. And even then the inferences will not be understood, since the only valuable foundation of all must be *metaphysic* truth, or none at all. It is with a view to furthering the study of the subject that we write suggestively. Much, however (we may add), will be found in the book to be very original. Some considerable proportion of its contents, we apprehend, as it will sufficiently startle, will be thought—certainly at first—to be beyond belief.

Lest it should be supposed that the author shares the opinions—apparently wholly realistic—of the writers who express their views in the Appendix, superadded at the end of the book, he is desirous of recording a firm disclaimer.

He admits, in many respects, the truth of *facts* put forward, whilst he dissents from, and disallows, as founded upon too hasty judgment and upon mistake, the conclusions which seem to be sought to be elicited from them. The object of the author in the present book is metaphysical *construction*, not religious *destruction*.

HARGRAVE JENNINGS.

CHAPTER I.

*Religion is to be found alone with its justification and
explanation in the relations between the sexes.   There and
therein only.*   To imply that the thing " Natural Selection,"
which can only arise, as any movement forward can arise,
through some power, or through something analogous to
the operation of the sexes, in choice and selection ; and
power upon that choice and selection to multiply, and to
bring into life, and to propagate like sexes, producing of
themselves; to imply that this thing, " Natural Selection" or the " survival of the fittest," is acting within the
matter, so to say, is, when argued rigidly down to foundation results, to say that " Natural Selection" is Deity
itself—which begs the whole question.

Such is inevitably the fate of all the logical methods of
philosophising, the Aristotelian or Baconian method,
which argues from particulars to generals; this is the
scientific, and the plausible way, but it is, as we have
always contended, the *wrong* way.   Once grant the
premiss, and it is all over with the argument, because
the question is already begged, and settled, nor can
there be farther dispute.   This is easily shown in the
fallacy of beginning with any assumption, or by appro-
priating any particular ground or foundation to commence

B

upon. Thus, there must be some truth, or the abstraction, truth, *can* be fixed, and become recognisable in the human reason. We assume that the human reason can become an efficient, or the foundation for truth. From this comes the fatal metaphysical error of discovering the possibility of human reason in truth, and the converse of finding a ground of truth to build upon, in human reason. Such concession at once gives science, and gives to realism all that it needs; and will admit and pass, as undoubted, all the innumerable links of any interminable chain of argument, leading anywhere, when the first touch or link or the premiss—whatever it be—is acknowledged as authentic, and a veritable thing. We are only correct when we retire into cloudland with speculation, and at once deny the possibility of special truth, or abstract truth, or indeed any truth. "Truth" being *your* truth, or *my* truth, or any man's truth. Where can we find the standard?

We remember that, many years ago, Robert and William Chambers, of Edinburgh, in a review of the current philosophies, with an explanation of their varying characteristics, chose to criticise the disbelieving philosopher, David Hume, who seeks to expose the fallacy of that which is accepted as the clearest possible common sense and reason, namely, of the invariable tie of connexion between cause and effect, or the certainty of cause being followed by effect, and effect being preceded by a cause. They ended with a summing up which was very efficacious and trenchant as far as it went, and seemed to lay open the whole of this apparently obvious absurdity of the great rationalist. The orthodox brothers thought their epigrammatic disposal of the question, and their derisive wonder at it, complete and unanswerable; but to what, in reality, did it all amount? To an evasion, not a resolution of the difficulty. They stated that, when Hume arrived at the end of his finely-sifted, elaborate metaphysical conclusions, and came out, at last, with such a startling climax, he only truly, and in fact, arrived at a belief, himself, and that he, who was denying the very possibility of belief, "came to a belief that there was no belief." This was a flying jeer, a Parthian dart, of the brothers Chambers; we do not know whether any doubt of the soundness of their philosophy ever occurred to them. They evidently thought they were carrying off the philosophical colours in triumph, after the skirmish, and exposing the nonsense of disconcerted Hume. It never penetrated to the conviction of these self-satisfied commentators, guiding the public judgment as they thought, that they were not confuting Hume, but only effecting their retreat under the cover of a witticism. What was the fact? They were only mistaking an *emotion* for a belief. Hume did not "believe" that there was no connexion between cause and effect. He only felt an emotion, or persuasion—a distrust whether there was, or whether there could be, necessarily and abstractedly, any connexion between cause and effect.

These two distinctions, in fact, philosophically stand wide apart. It is only in the coarse metaphysical intellect that they are not kept separate. And most of the modern philosophers, because their philosophical intellects are not of the highest, and their penetration not of the refined character—nature having denied them the delicate power of analysis, or the closest discrimination, confound emotions of the heart with reasons and con-

clusions of the intellect and the head;—while, in fact,
the head and the heart, or the reason and the affections,
have been set in hopeless opposition to each other from
the beginning of time. Men believe, and yet cannot be
said to have faith. Men have faith (that is, know), and
yet cannot be said to believe. Thus men have faith in
what they cannot believe, for instance, in transubstantia-
tion. And they have belief in what they can never know,
that is, in the spiritual world, and in the doctrine of
spirits; and in past events, which, however, did not
certainly transact as related. There is, indeed, no "fact"
which cannot be argued away, and shown to be nothing.
Very consolatory this, for the inhabitants of that which
they presume is a real world. It has been shown, even,
conclusively, that it is impossible that man can be in
contact with real solidity; and that Time itself is only
an abstraction.

The purport of the foregoing remarks will be the more
readily seen as we advance with our theme, and recognise
the religious intensity of the Phallic worship, its vitality,
and its display in the Phallic monuments, both in those
devoted to the solar and the lunar myths, which equally
indicate the same Fire-Worship in its grand division of
celestial and terrestrial adoration. In this element of
"Fire" and the magical rites and formulæ arising out of
it, all the mystic analysis and anatomy of Nature rest:
and this science is genuine, as founded on the astronomy
and astrology of the Chaldeans and other early nations,
who were the heirs of the first knowledge or revelation.

CHAPTER II.

THE HISTORY OF THE PHALLIC "SYMBOL-STRUCTURES;"
THEIR ORIGIN, GENEALOGY, AND VARIETY THROUGH
THE SUCCESSION OF THE HISTORICO-RELIGIOUS AGES.

To cite the expressions of a very able and original
writer, who adopted the subject of Phallicism, and the
highly important part it has played in the history of
the religions of the world, we might have spoken of
the terms in which we treat of our general subject, in
the present chapter. We might have professed to give
'The Causes of the Original Dispersion of Primitive
Nations in times of remote antiquity;' and enlarged on
' presumptive proofs of original connexion between
various -nations, now widely scattered; deducible from a
critical examination into the intrinsic signification and
character of ancient sacred edifices, &c., of which the
ruins and imperishable remains still exist in several
countries.' This was substantially the title of an ably
reasoned article, published under the name of ΠΡΩΤΕΥΣ,
author of a work on the "Real Nature of the Sin of
Adam." The article appeared with the two words,
"Fiat Lux," printed on its forefront, in the *Freemasons'
Quarterly Review*, in the year 1840. In proceeding with
this dissertation the author says he shall discuss the
subject generally, under the four following heads—viz. :
Firstly, in examining what was in reality intended, mystically figured, and represented, under the colossal and
other national monuments, and sacred edifices of antiquity.

—*Secondly*, in showing that it was in consequence of a disturbance which took place in the unity of the faith of the early inhabitants of the earth, at the renewed period of its existence (that is to say, soon after the Flood), that these same symbolical edifices came to be erected in commemoration of the grand schismatic division.— *Thirdly*, in setting forth that the ancient emigrations with which we are acquainted, are to be distinctly attributed, in the first instance, solely to this division of faith and to separate religious opinions.—*Fourthly*, and chiefly, in pointing out the value of a system of interpretation which seems to supply the only key for expounding the religious mysteries of all nations, or which may prevail to open the sealed historic volume that contains the records of remote antiquity, and by applying it to the problematical dispersion of nations, (which has so often occupied the attention of the learned), and tracing the original motives of their separation by a series of almost irrefutable inferences, show that it may thus be determined on a surer basis than can otherwise be established, what nations were in reality of an original stock, by proving them to have held common religious opinions when, as yet, but two grand sectarian divisions disputed for ascendency in the minds of men.

In answer to the first of these inquiries, as to what was mystically figured, and represented under the colossal and other monuments and sacred edifices of antiquity, we will proceed to designate respectively, as the head and type of all succeeding edifices of like character, the Tower of Babel, and the great Pyramids of Egypt. The first of these was erected not long after the foundation of the Chaldæan monarchy, by Nimrod, the son of Cush, 2221 B.C.

The temple of Belus formed a square nearly three miles in compass. In the middle of the temple was an immense tower, six hundred feet in height. The ruins are now two hundred and thirty-five feet high. The Great. Pyramid forms a square, each side of whose base is seven hundred and forty-five feet, and covers an area of nearly fourteen acres. The perpendicular height is five hundred and sixty feet. The Pyramids were erected probably not long after the foundation of the Egyptian monarchy by Misraim, the son of Ham, 2188 B.C., Babylon and Memphis being among the first cities built after the Flood. And when the totally different *forms* of these immense national edifices are considered, the inquiring mind can scarcely fail to seek for the causes which decided their ancient architects to employ so gigantic a mass of materials, in one or the other of these two definite forms, above every other which might have been selected; and we think it will scarcely be denied that the forms respectively of these stupendous monuments (which, as will be shown, were only the original archetypes of innumerable others which have been subsequently constructed,) must unavoidably be considered as having been adopted as the carrying out of some paramount idea or intention on the part of their primeval founders.

There is cause to believe, that in the erection of the Chaldæan Tower, the principles of true " Masonry" were at first abided by; but, subsequently, the corruption of human nature urging men to overthrow a spiritual worship, which absolutely required purity and holiness, they sought to establish a system that virtually inculcated the worship of the creature more than the Creator, and furnished a pretext for the practice of unrestrained licentiousness, as part and parcel of religious rites. Such was the ancient worship of the *Lingam*—a worship which we read of as recognised and established throughout all antiquity; such was the object really worshipped under its colossal representative, in the Chaldæan Tower, that magnificent, monster "Upright," defiant, as it were, or appealing, for both of these meanings are, in certain senses, (and acceptations), identical. This was the prodigious Tower, or obelis*c*, (or obelis*k*, the "k" and the "c" being interchangeable), known from the description in Scripture, and the hints contained in its allegories, or rather magnificent myths, as to the causes of the original Dispersion, as the Tower of Babel, Bab, or Babble. Thence has come down to us the name for vain talking, confusion, the "confusion of tongues," or languages; when the sudden supernatural interposition came from the divine Architect of the Universe, making a fool of mankind, and, in the impossibility of the people understanding each other's meaning, rendering society, or a general community of design and purpose of the human race, as working to one common end—however obvious, in common sense, the object might be—*impossible.*

We are here seeking to establish, firstly, the philosophical possibility of magic; and, secondly, the actual working of magic in the real affairs of the world; notwithstanding the contradictions of common sense, rightly enough, perhaps, to the possibility of magic, which means the unnatural interference with nature, and is a contradiction in terms, when we estimate "nature" as all that is, or as fixed and unalterable, in its own laws, as supreme; especially, in the total absence of any proof, at any time, or at any period of the world's history, as receivable in record or testimony, reasonable and believable, that anything like magic, or interference from without nature, ever obtruded or interjected from outside that nature, *into* that nature—which, however mistaken or misunderstood from the natural infirmities of man—still "builds the world," and *is* the world:—nothing other being so, or being possible to be so. But, after all— man is not all! Nor is common sense all—or indeed *anything* out of this our world of Man!

So much for this famous Chaldæan Tower, "Tower of Babel," or PHALLUS, of whose notorious existence traditions, even in the most remote nations, almost universally exist; and of whose actual signification many weighty proofs have been collected by that very zealous, penetrating and able antiquary, the late Mr. Henry O'Brien, author of a very conclusive book, "The Round Towers of Ireland." These Round Towers were all "Phalli," or· Fire-Towers, raised in adherence to, and in expression of the inconceivably ancient faith of the Persians, Parsees, or Fire-worshippers. To Mr. O'Brien's proofs we might certainly add others equally numerous and irrefragable, were we here intending, in this chapter, an elaborate treatise, instead of a circumscribed review of the circumstances affording proofs.

The worship of the Lingam, then, of which the *Pillar Tower* was, as has been said, a gigantic figure, involved and signified the worship of the Male Principle of the Universe; by which was intended, originally, as has been intimated, the worship of the True and Only God; in accordance with which assertion we find that one interpretation of the word Jehovah undoubtedly signifies the Universal Male. In India, where undeniable proofs have been found of the existence, at one period, of true "Masonry" (see *Freemasons' Quarterly Review*, p. 159), this signification is found to be involved in the names of the principal deities. Accordingly we find that temples in honour of this Universal Male Power, were always erected in the figure of its representative, the Lingam; that is to say, in the form of a tower or column—God in his unity. Almost innumerable examples of such edifices abound in ancient countries, where this worship was either primitive, or introduced at later periods, and they fully illustrate these facts.

Wilford remarks (*Works*, vol. iii., 365) that the Phallus was publicly worshipped by the name of Balleswara Linga, on the banks of the Euphrates. The cubic room in the cave of Elephanta likewise contains the Lingam (vol. iv., 413), as does also the pagoda of stone at Maherbaliporam, or City of the Great Baal (vol. v., 69). Sir William Jones observes, (vol. ii., 47), " columns were erected, perhaps as gnomons, others probably to represent the Phallus of Iswara." Enough has here been cited, without doubt, to dispose both the learned and the unlearned to consider that the true signification of the pillar and tower was in reality such as has here been stated.

In many parts of the Bible we find the pillar to have been undoubtedly a sacred emblem; as in *Isaiah*, xix. : " In that day shall there be an altar to Jehovah in the midst of the land of Egypt, and a *pillar* at the border thereof, to Jehovah, and it shall be for *a sign*, and a *witness to the Lord.*" And this was the especial form in which it pleased God himself to appear, when he dwelt in the pillar that went before his chosen people, as solemnly recorded by Moses.

When, however, pillars were set up to receive the profane rites of idolatrous worship, we find them noticed in Scripture as an abomination, in like manner as their great Babylonian archetype; which being obnoxious to God, as such, was destroyed by "fire from Heaven," as its blasted and vitrified ruins still remain incontrovertibly to attest.

Having thus briefly noticed the worship of the LINGAM, or male principle, it remains to show what was the true and real thing signified under the form of the PYRAMID, TRIANGLE, or CONE: and with respect to the mysteries concealed and represented in the figure of the pyramid, I apprehend, that before Mr. O'Brien's luminous remarks on that subject, the scientific world in general were in almost Cimmerian obscurity as to the real and opposite tendency of the worship indicated by edifices erected in that form. A remark in the *Asiatic Researches* (vol. ii., 477), that "the pyramids of Egypt, as well as those discovered in Ireland, [the Round Towers are meant, which are *obelisks*, and not *pyramids*], and probably, too, the Tower of Babel, seem to have been intended as nothing more than images of Mahadeo,"* shows how confused were the notions of the learned, as to the real character of the pyramid, "when we are thus led to suppose that the *pyramid* and *tower* alike represent an identical and male power, and typify an identical object of adoration." The writer of the foregoing passages seems to be in some fault here, because the pyramids, towers, obelisks, and pillars, although of the same family of objects, imply a different significance. In reality, the towers and inclined pillars, and the obelisks with the

* *Mahadeo*, Maha-Deo—How like, this, to "Mother of God!"

characteristic which the architects call the "orbicular" curve, are the same as the broad pyramid, only slim and aspiring; and the pyramids are the same as the pillars and towers, only broad in the base and latitudinal. The fact of the matter is that all of these are pyramidal forms, and that they only differ in their slimness or breadth, for they all express the same religious, mysterious idea ; which is, swelling, rising, or extension— the characteristic or the motive movement, in both sexes, for that "grand act"—that grand human act—which secures us everything, the uprising and protrusion of the peculiar instruments, male and female, for success in the sexual magic congress. This we shall declare in different parts of our book, to be MAGIC, and a holy sacrament or charm ; and it doubtless is sympathetic magnetism of its kind, from which it is perfectly possible, and proper, to extract all irregular ideas, or obscenity, if the mind be purified adequately to will it so.

Certain philosophers have chosen to view this matter in another light, in regard of the sameness of the Phallic symbols, whether the pillar, tower, or pyramid. We reckon all these symbol-structures to signify, ultimately, but one thing—the "Fire," apotheosised as celestial, and worshipped as the only possible, and the genuine representative of the supreme, the chief deity, to be addressed in adoration, appeased and moved to mercy in mystic rites, protesting sacrifices, and innumerable appealing services, solemnities and observances, forming a fixed code, constituting an immutable law; to be confided to the hand of the Arch-Priests as Sovereigns, and to Sovereigns in their character of Hierophants and Sacred Guardians. These theorists say that as the tower was sacred to the male power of the universe, so likewise was the pyramid, triangle, or cone, adopted by the votaries of an opposite worship, as the real and consecrated emblem and representation of that procreative female energy in which, according to them (considering it as the true and vital conceptive power of nature), resided absolutely and solely the underived principle of life ; which female power they chose alone to deify, and, like their opponents, consecrated their unhallowed worship by the most profane and licentious rites.

Thus the great Pyramids were at Memphis the colossal monuments of a separate worship, with all its concomitant mysteries ; and as in the Tower of Babel, the threefold objects of astronomy, astrology, and religion were indissolubly involved and united in them.

Baron Humboldt observes, in his *Researches* (in total ignorance, however, of this theory), " In every part of the globe, on the ridge of the Cordilleras as well as in the Isle of Samothrace, in the Ægean Sea, fragments of primitive languages are preserved in religious rites." Sir William Jones expressly states that the meaning of ' *yóni*' or ' *bhaga*,' is undoubtedly the female special sensual part ; and in his plate of the Hindu Lunar Mansions, (see the article on the Antiquity of the Indian Zodiac), this constellation of the ' yóni' is figured as three stars, inclosed by the Hindu draughtsman in a representation of *that object ;* which, in his figure, is made to resemble an inverted pyramid, or truncated cone. Venus Genetrix is sometimes represented in the form of a conical marble ; "for the reason of which figure," says Tacitus, " we are left in the dark ;" but, adds Sir William Jones, " the reason appears too clearly in the temples and paintings of

Hindustan, where it never seems to have entered the heads of the legislators or people, that anything *natural* could be offensively indecent." Wilford mentions that according to Theodoret, Arnobius, and Clemens Alexandrinus, the Yoni of the Hindus was the sole object of veneration in the mysteries of Eleusis. For proofs of the high antiquity of this worship in China, the discerning reader need only consult Lord Macartney's *Travels*, vol. i. 'Hager, Monument of Yu.' "In both *Americas*," we learn, "it is a matter of inquiry what was the intention of the natives when they raised so many artificial pyramidal hills, several of which appear to have served neither as tombs, nor watch-towers, nor the base of a temple." About 2,000 years before our era, sacrifices were offered in China, to the supreme being, on four great mountains, called the Four Yo. The whole country of Mexico abounded in pyramids, and Humboldt declares the basis of the Great Cholula to have been twice as broad as that of the Egyptian Cheops, though its height is little more than that of Mycerinus. The fact is, that wherever this peculiar worship has flourished (and it must never be lost sight of that all idolatry can be shown to have been originally based on one or other ramification of it,) traces are left behind and relics remain, which have always been found to puzzle the learned antiquarian no less than the unlettered conjecturer.

"In the Mexican Codex Borgianus," says Humboldt, "the head of the sacrificing priest is covered with one of those conical caps which are worn in China and on the north-west coast of America; opposite this figure is seated the god of fire." We may note that the triangle was indisputably a sacred emblem from all antiquity, as might be shown by innumerable examples. There are exceedingly curious coins called *Cistophori* of Pergamos, which city Cicero mentions as possessing a great number of them, on which we see represented various, devices, indicative of recondite mysteries; the triangle surmounting the whole, and held in the deadly fangs of serpents.

In commenting on the particular branch of idolatry under discussion, we cannot but remark, that there appears just reason to believe, that this was *the peculiar abomination* into which the Ten Tribes of Israel lapsed, at their separation from Judah under Jeroboam. Indeed strong presumptive proof is offered, insomuch as, from the account given by Herodotus, and cited by Josephus, of the invasion of the Egyptian Shishak, under Rehoboam, it appears that, having conquered Jerusalem, and *defiled the public buildings*, by carving on them the distinctive symbols of his own peculiar and national creed (that is to say, according to the same author, by defacing them with *representations of that very symbol, the mysterious yóni*, which we have been discussing), he returned to his own country without in any way molesting Samaria, the residence of the Ten Tribes, who, it needs not any great measure of sagacity to perceive, had doubtless embraced his religious views. What those views were, in the sight of God, is fully expressed in *Kings,* 1, xiv., 7, 8, 9, and xv., 26, 30, 34; also *Kings,* 2, iii., 2, 3, &c.

It is supposed by those who have pursued these deeply interesting and original Phallic inquiries the most closely, and achieved philosophic results therefrom with the greatest success, that it was in consequence of a disturbance which took place in the unity of the faith of the early inhabitants of the earth, that is to say, soon after the Flood, that these same symbolical edifices came to be erected, in commemoration of the grand schismatic division.

At the time of the building of Babel, we have the highest authority for knowing that the sentiments of the men then and there engaged, were in complete unison, for Moses records that "the Lord said, Behold, the people is One." Had this unity of feeling been manifested in persevering in the worship of the true and only God, upon whose almighty name men already began to call, even while Adam was yet alive, doubtless it would have been, instead of a subject of reproach, an occasion of approval to Him "whose name is One." (See *Ephes.*, iv., 5, 6.) But when this unanimity was manifested only in the departure of men from the principles of religion and true 'Masonry,' and consequently from Truth itself, the Lord God "scattered them abroad," as we read, "upon the face of all the earth."

As has been already observed, traditions are still extended almost throughout the length and breadth of the earth, of this miraculous and notable transaction: it is impossible in the space here assigned even casually to designate the various and modified forms in which this history has been handed down, from the remarkable legend preserved by the Mexican priests, as related by Humboldt, even to the wild fables believed by the savages of the South Seas, and strangely analogous to the primeval account.

In Wilford's *Essay on the Nile*, vol. iii., p. 360, we find that this diversity of opinion (*i.e.* the superiority of the male or female emblem of the sexual part, that of generation, in regard of the idolatrous, magic worship) seems to have occasioned the general war which is often mentioned in the Puranas, and was celebrated by the poets of the west as the basis of the Grecian mythology. According to both Nonnus and the Hindu mythologists, it began in India, whence it spread over the whole globe, and all mankind appear to have borne a part in it. These physiological contests, arising from a profound considera- tion of the mysteries of animal generation, and its super- natural "wherefore," and on the comparative influences of the sexes in the production of perfect offspring (in itself, down to this instant day, the greatest possible, and the apparently irresolvable, mystery):—these mighty physiological disputes, induced in the reflective wisdom of the earliest thinkers, laid the sublime foundations of the Phallic Worship. They led to violent schisms in religion, and even to bloody and devastating wars, which have wholly passed out of the history of these earliest times ; or rather they have never been recorded in history; remaining only as a tradition, or, if at all holding place, holding it only in the faintest, although the sublimest form, as a *fable*. These physiological contests were dis- guised under a veil of the wildest allegories and emblems, in Egypt, and India especially, and generally in every other country.

The epoch of warfare and bloodshed is alluded to frequently as the " Age of Contention," or " Confusion." That this essential difference of opinion as to the real ascendency and superiority of *male* or *female*, as such, involved also the physical problem of the predominant agency of either sex in the mystery of generation, which it is clear they were pleased erroneously to look upon as synonymous with Creation itself, is we think fully evident.

c

We are inclined, however, also to believe that the Pish-de-Danaan sect, those fierce contenders for the supremacy of the female influence, certainly derived no little of the plausibility of their pretensions from a reference to the primeval prophecy that the " WOMAN's seed should bruise the serpent's head."   In that sense at least it is natural to suppose that they could hardly fail to consider otherwise than as supremely sacred and magical, that mystical centre of woman's body, reference to which is, in the grandly superstitious and grandly sacramental sense, made in a whisper, the best proof of the possibility of magic, and of the supernatural, motived, directly personal interference of the gods (by whatever name we may call Them, or, in concentration, as One, Him) with the doings of Man.   That female part, before which we even, now, apart from Phallicism, can "fall down and worship," as the most glorious object in all God's creation, when disclosed as the Rose in the Garden of Flowers in the perfectly-formed naked* figure of a beautiful woman, is, in fact, that which it is desecration to uncover other than reverentially and worthily.   Notably, according to the ancient true ideas, especially among the Jews, it was

---

* The word "naked," considered radically, comes, we think, from the Greek word—" Nike"—meaning " victory," in one sense as the victory of the Evil Genius, and also " victory" in the sense of power—that is, female power. The same word also signifies "death." Thus in *Genesis :—*

" But of the fruit of the tree which is in the midst of the Garden, God hath said :—'Ye shall not eat of it, neither shall ye touch it— LEST YE DIE !' " This injunction, be it remarked, strangely and contradictorily as it sounds, was made to both " Man" and " Woman."— (*Genesis.*—Chap. iii., v. 3.) The whole of Genesis is cabalistic, and therefore of the fullest force, though its purpose and its meanings are impenetrably covered over with mystery.

always regarded as the very centre and most sacred point of the religions. Amongst the Hebrews it was philosophically and mystically considered as deep sunk in the profundities of mystery, to break in, unpreparedly, upon which would impugn the eternal supernatural " charm" the legend of which lay inextricably in the " Cabala :" and which display would compromise, nay, obliterate its purpose and use, in the reproduction of the generations ; thus disobeying, in its extinguishment, the enjoined exercise of the physical means for the renewal and perpetuation of life out of ourselves. The abstract strangeness of this fact has escaped the wonder of people, however startling it would appear of itself, even naturally, except from experience, which takes away the surprise from everything, and which familiarity reconciles us to the miracle even of our own being.

Take away the shame incident to the sexual parts of woman and of man, and accustom us to the continual familiar sight of them, and we shall grow to regard them with as much indifference as the face or the feet. Shame, human shame, is taught and acquired, it being the effect of community, coming from the natural habit of blushing at fellowship in relation to these things. We never blush at the mere consciousness of being in love, yet grow confused even at love which is the purest when we are brought to book in the sight of other people. Another remarkable effect in the case of experiencing passion, or love, is that when it is felt most intensely, it becomes embodied, as it were, even as a sort of sickness. And it is doubtful whether, indeed, to the natural man, love be not a disease, like a fever that is caught, although it is delicious in its sensations, and in its " love-lorn" weakness and lassitude.　Is this a proof of what strange, glorious, unimaginable heaven there may be prepared for us, of which, in this state, we know nothing; when even its premonitory, anticipative, mysterious illnesses, or diseases, may be actually the deliciously divine affliction of immortal Love, descending out of the skies, or out of the celestial regions, into the responsive soul of man? Thus it may really be profoundly true, as Plato thought, that not only the "music of the spheres is true," and that, thus, music is veritably the atmosphere, or magnetism, of the angels, as Robert Flood and the Rosicrucians taught; but that Shakespeare was right when he implied that "*Music* is the food of love;" which almost every man's and woman's daily experience assures them it must be.

We were, however, about to instance, as a remarkable proof of the purifying power of real, intense, although personal love, when gone forth and incorporate, as it were, into the object, which then becomes truly an enchanted object, that, in these exalted cases, *bodily desire* for the object is rarely felt or thought of,* which would seem to show, wild enough as it seems to assert it, that

* If it be thought about at all, in relation to the individual with whom the person may be in love, in these exalted cases, the thought of the "loved one" is simply magic *in excelsis*, or a state of passionate delirium, in which the object transcends out of the natural. Hence Platonic love, and love of the highest, may be true. Therefore this sort of love is so refined and spiritual as to be sinless, bodily contact being impossible of it. Such ideas as the foregoing are the groundwork and the *raison d'être* of the possibility of perfect monasticism; and of nunhood or the maintenance of perpetual virginity; and of the realisation of that self-devoted trampling upon the flesh, which is the glorious distinctive mark of the Saints, Martyrs, and Hermits, male and female, all the more gloriously great, when the one class—as in the Roman

the passion of copulation is truly accidental to man, and not natural to him. [Refer to our chapter upon the Mystic Anatomy of Henry Cornelius Agrippa, and to passages referring to the reveries of some of the Gnostics.] Indeed, unless the mystery maintained in the hiding away and rendering unknown these objects had conserved completely the irresistible desire to " know," and to be secret viewers of the male special distinctions and the female special peculiarities—the human man, having a soul, and woman, having a soul, as a son and a daughter of God in a certain sublime, physical sense—it would seem philosophically that desire must have become obliterated, and that means must have failed, through the extinguishment, first of impulse, and then absolutely of power—the magic, in this respect, being conjured out of man through interference, *ab extra;* with the fullest proof of concentrate, occasional design of a still stronger magic, and of a still more powerful exertion of power than the congenital magic and the natural power. For it must always be remembered that man is an object of himself, as a being with a " soul," shipwrecked from without (he knows not whence), into this world of animated forms, with destinies wholly opposite ; and here produced and domesticated wholly for a different object, seemingly by accident, as a contrast and phenomenon, the ruin of a ruined spirit, perhaps, yet the acknowledged master, no mate, of all the lower animals, even up to those of the highest grade, whose characteristics yet touch the brute

Catholic religion they are presumed to be—are perfect, and the other class, the female devotees, are beautiful. All this, from a certain point of view, is considered fanaticism ; but nevertheless it is a very fine fanaticism.

in some respects. Some such view as this is clearly the only hope of humanity. Man is a machine, dependent upon the surrounding elements, and upon his food and its decomposition for his nutrition, and consuming his exquisitely-attuned and manipulated machinery, gradually, in the terrestrial, vital, animal heat (or " flameless fire," to make use of a paradoxical figure) ; for man falls to pieces (again, a figure or rhodomontade), when he can no longer maintain himself in his " nature." Yet the valorous defence, that his nature makes, even against itself, is truly wonderful, stupendous. But man fails, at last, in the incessant war, because he is endowed—however, in health and constitution, richly endowed—only to endure for a brief time. There is a never-ceasing ravage, except for the indispensable intervals of restoring sleep, effected upon his fine nerves ; upon which his emotions, beautiful, or the reverse, according to his refinement, play as upon harpstrings, when the angels touch or the devils assail. All this, the astrologers say, is regulated by the " traverse through time" of his horoscope (fatality, or necessity) ; although man, nevertheless, has his independent will, or power of election for good or evil, in ways and by methods which supernaturally render free-will and " necessity" identical in the divine counsels ; of which Man, in his extremely limited capacity, " most ignorant of what he's most assured," can form no more conclusive idea, than he can of abstract time or space, or anything scarcely, even the " cogito, ergo sum," identity. He has only a fear of that outside—and a reverence for it, born out of fear, scarcely out of love of it.

CHAPTER III.

THE STORY OF THE CLASSES OF THE PHALLI.

THE two influences, Male and Female, are conspicuous in certain differences in the Phallic monuments, which unitedly, however, signify the same thing. The disputes of the comparative superiority of the Male over the Female principle, or of the Female over the Male, were the origin, amongst the earliest nations, of vast desolating wars, of which no history, scarcely even legend, has descended to modern periods. Therefore, no account remains of these primeval wars, which brought about the building of the famous Tower of Babel, and were ultimately the cause of the confusion of languages and the original dispersion of the nations. Obelisks, Towers, and Steeples represent and figure forth the Male principle. Pyramids, Circular magnified forms, and Rhomboidal, or Undulating, Serpentine shapes, denote the Female natural power. The one set of forms are masculine; therefore aggressive, and compelling. The other set of forms are feminine; therefore submissive, and ennobling. But all are alike Phallic, and mean the same thing, that is the natural motived power which causes and directs the world, that power which *is* the world, in fact.

We have perhaps brought sufficiently into view, and realised to the reader's attention, as most important, in every sense, as explanatory of religion and of religious mysteries, both the theories of the myths, and the actualities of the mysteries, whether heathen or ethnic,

Christian or vindicatory. These Phallic objects, innumerable, are always peculiar in their form, and are of all
sizes. If these sometimes prodigious structures are
Obelisks, Columns, or Pillars, or as occasionally happens,
single, rough-hewn, or partly-fashioned uprights, they
represent and figure forth the male principle. Subsequent to the very early, devotional ages, these pins, or
uprights, assumed the forms of solid or slender towers,
tors, or springing, rising, pointed fabrics. Amongst the
Muslemmim these were minarets, with egg-shaped sum-
mits; in the architectural practice among the Christians,
the tower attenuated into the spire or steeple. But the
memorial structures with the larger base, and with that
broader incidence which might be denominated, with a
certain aptness, the Saturnian angle, indicated the opposite influence, that of the Female, in mystic type or
apotheosis. These symbol-structures, involving the idea
of the feminine power, are the more broadly vaulting in
shape. Chief, and most majestic of all these monuments,
are the Pyramids. All the mystical monuments of this
form and fashion are in the general sense, equally Phalli—
that is, devoted to, and in witness of the worship of the
distinctive sexual peculiarities. We accept the whole as
meaning the one thing, Phallicism, all interpreted under the
general, rising, forceful form, aspiring towards the stars.
Stately beyond idea, and gloomily majestic, as is the aspect
of these Lunar or Womanly monumental structures, they
can be soon distinguished. This group of the Feminine-
Phallic forms comprises the Pyramids in the first rank.
The Obelisk is a shrunken, vertically thin, concentrated
pyramid: the Pyramid is a widely squared out obelisk:
both express the same idea. In the conveyance of certain

ideas to those who contemplate them, the pyramid boasts of prouder significance, and impresses with a hint of still more impenetrable and more removed mystery. We seem to gather dim, supernatural ideas of the mighty mother of Nature, the dusk divinity crowned with towers, the ancientest among the ancients, the Isis, or mysterious consort of the Dethroned, and Ruined, that almost two-sexed entity without a name, She of the Veil which is never to be lifted, perhaps not even by the angels, for their knowledge is limited. In short, this tremendous abstraction, Cybele, *Ideæ Mater*, Isiac controller of the zodiacs, whatever she be, has her representative figure in the half-buried Sphynx, even to our own day, watching the stars, although nearly swallowed up in the engulphing sands. This is the Gorgon survival of the period of the Ark, eldest daughter of the mythologies, whose other face (for, Janus-like, she looks two ways,) turned away from the world, is beautiful as the fairest one of Paradise. That other face of the Gorgon, or Sphynx, resembles, in one respect, that side of the Lunar disc; the side of the Moon turned away from observers on the earth, that face which no mortal eye ever saw, or will see, and which, for this reason, is one of the greatest mysteries in all the sky.

The foregoing remarks furnish the clue to this double history of the Phallus, in the divided character of its worship, whether the Obelisk or Pillar, or whether the Pyramid be the idol. It is too plain to be misunderstood. As the Greeks wrote *Palai* for Páli, they rendered the word Paliputra, by *Palaigonos*, which also means the offspring of Páli, literally signifying the offspring of the Phallus. It was notoriously the *Yóni* and not the *Phallus*, which alone received the veneration of the Hindus, though now divided into innumerable sects and an inextricable maze of polytheism. Wilford observes that the Yávanas were the ancestors of the Greeks, and (vol. iii., p. 358) that the Pandits insist that the words *Yávana* and *Yóni* are derived from the same root, *Yu*, and that the Yávanas were so named from their obstinate assertion of a superior influence in the female over the male nature. An ancient book on astronomy, in Sanscrit, bears the title of *Yávana Jàtica*, which may be interpreted "the Ionic sect." There is an ancient proverb amongst the Pandits, that "no base creature can be lower than a Yávana," truly showing the fluctuating nature of human opinions and theories, which, nevertheless, have torn the bosom of society, and shaken nations to their centre. Their creed caused the new people in Greece to name their new country itself Ionia, from that consecrated Yóni which they revered, and to distinguish themselves as the Ionic, or Yó-nic sect, in indubitable reference to their peculiar opinions. These and such-like researches, furnish us with the real meaning of proper names, and amongst others that of the great goddess Ju-no, which Wilford asserts to be derived from the Yóni of the Hindus; also if we analyse the name of Diana, or Di-Yana, the great goddess of the Ephesians, we shall at once perceive an identical etymology; and when we remember that Ju-no was fabled to have been born at Argos, and that she was peculiarly worshipped *there*, we shall fully coincide in that opinion, for it is to be observed that this name of Argha is derived from the Bhaga of the Hindus, and both signified the Yóni, and likewise an ark or boat, which was used throughout antiquity as a type of the Yóni itself. The Hindu goddess, Bagis, was indifferently called Vagis, from which, no doubt, is derived the Latin *vagina;* and when we remember that Plutarch makes the otherwise inexplicable assertion, that Osiris* (or the incarnation of the male principle) was commander of the Argo; and when we learn that the true meaning of the name Argha-nát'ha, or, as we mostly render it, (speaking of the great idol), Jagernath, is no other than "lord of the boat," we shall perceive at once the drift of these dark sentences, when truly and intelligibly expounded.

The discussion of this word *Argha* naturally induces us to remark concerning an intermediate or middle sect, which, says Wilford, "is now prevalent in India, and which was generally diffused over ancient Europe." It was introduced by the Pelargi, who, Herodotus says, were the same as the Pelasgi. Many ancient writers affirm that they were one of the most ancient peoples in the world. It is asserted that they first inhabited Argolis, and about 1883, B.C., passed into Œmonia, or Yomonia, and were afterwards dispersed, or emigrated into several parts of Greece. Some of the Pelasgians that had been driven from Attica, (Yà-tica), settled at Lemnos, whither, some time after, they carried some Athenian women, whom they had seized on the coast of Africa. They raised children by these captive females, but afterwards destroyed them together with their mothers, through jealousy, because they differed in manners from themselves, which horrid murder was attended by a dreadful pestilence. Such is the account given by the classic writers (Pausanias, Strabo, Herodotus, Plato,

* *Osiris* and *Isis,* the *Is'wara* and *I'si* of the Hindus.

Virgil, Ovid, Flaccus, Seneca, &c.). But, when we weigh the foregoing arguments, can we doubt that these women were destroyed through jealousy of their religion, and not because they differed merely in manners, in accordance with the peculiar characteristics of fanaticism, which brooks no opposition to its devouring nature?

The word Pelargos was derived, says Wilford, from P'hala and Argha, (Phallus, and Argha from Bhaga, or Yóni), those mysterious types which the later mythologist distinguished under the names of Pallas and Argo.

The Pelargi venerated both male and female principles in union, as their compound appellation indicates, and represented them conjointly, when their powers were supposed to be combined, by the intersection of two equilateral triangles, thus, ×, that peculiar symbol

" Form'd all mysteries to bear,"

the emblem of Lux, and to which innumerable perfections and virtues, including those of the Cross, have been attributed, from time immemorial. The union of these two symbols, denoting the Male nature, and the Female nature, or the Phallus, the mark of which is the *upright* line, and the Yoni, the recognitive mark of which is the *horizontal* line, are best rendered, or depicted, in the double, or conjoined equilateral triangle in intersection. The pyramidal, aspiring, equilateral triangle is Male, and signifies Fire, and the rushing force of fire, mounting upwards in its own impulse, contradicting nature, inasmuch as it shoots up against gravity. The pyramid in reverse, or pointing down, is the indicating symbol of Water, or of the lunar, Female influence. The cross section of these all-significant figures gives the sexalpha,

or Six-Alphas, the one half of the Cabalistic Machataloth
or the six ascending signs of the zodiac, moving to junction upwards in their influences (the one half of the
ecliptic, figuratively the spear or glaive of Saint Michael),
and also the other half of the same, six signs in reverse,
meaning the junction, in cross action, and importing the
whole number of the astronomical, and astrological, twelve
equal divisions, or the Twelve Signs of the Great Circle.
This, also, means the dominion of the Moon in man's
body, as passing through all the twelve signs. The
symbol, or sign, of this mystical union is framed as
thus :—Fire-Water, Water-Fire, Male-Female, Female-
Male, in equal interchange, and the figure representing its
idea, its glyph or special "hieroglyph," is given in our
illustration. This figure means Life mystically, and the
giving of life; it is the solemn mark, typical of the sexes in
conjunction ; and it is also called the seal of the princely
magician, Solomon, the King of the Jews, who builds and
sanctifies the temple, Solomon's temple ; the myths regarding which are manifold. Solomon, in this view, is not only
the monarch, and the mighty enchanter ; he is not only the
king of the Jews, but he is, also, supernaturally viewed,
the Champion, or Hero of the Fire. Fire, in all the
religions, has been chosen as the representative mark of
the supreme divinity, as the most faithful and closest
mystical celestial image ; as that idea of God vouchsafed
and approved ; in all the forms of faith, Chaldaic, Hebrew,
Oriental, Egyptian, Greek, Roman, Northern and Southern, Eastern and Western, nay, distinguishing the
Mexican and Peruvian, the Toltecque, and other religions
found prevailing on the discovery of the New World;
and all which, heathen and Christian alike, find direct

exemplification in the Phalli, speaking as it were all over the world, from all time; and yet remaining the symbol (only to be understood by the " Rosicrucians," and even to these vouchsafed, limitedly, with the " seven-fold guard" for silence,) which gives to Man, mystically and supernaturally, at once his only hope and, at the same time, his deepest dread. For, according to the assertion of the ancient philosopher, man found all his Gods in *fear*.

With the analysis of one more example we must imperfectly conclude this portion of our Gnostic subject; and the next example that occurs in this line of examination is the history of Mycenæ; which, we are of opinion, will confirm what has hitherto been advanced. Mycenæ, on which *name* Henry O'Brien has commented, was situate at the extremity of the plain of Argos, and was the capital of a kingdom whose last sovereign, Epytus, was dispossessed, 1104, B.C., on the return of the Heraclidæ, descendants of Hercules.

History informs us that Hercules was a Mycenæan prince, who was, for some reason or other, banished with all his family and descendants from the country, and his throne possessed by an usurper. Let us examine this name of Hercules. Chris, becoming the Christus, Christ, in the Christian ideas, or the Conservator, Saviour, the Greeks used to express by × or Spanish *iota*, the aspirated *ha* of the Orientals, who said *haris*. In Hebrew, *heres* signifies the Sun (Isaiah, xix. 18), but in Arabic the meaning of the radical word is to *preserve* (*haris, preserver*); and Heri-cal, from which Hercules, is a Hindoo name of the sun. " I cannot help suspecting," says Wilford, " that Hercules is the same with *Heracula*, and signifying the race of Hera or Heri ;" that is, the children of the sun, of which the Phallus always presented the emblem, as the vivifier and preserver of nature. Hence, perhaps, the cry, or appeal, Haro! (Rescue! Preserve!) in Jersey. This is valid by ancient law. We may here observe, as a curious citation, that this is a very old custom in Jersey, surviving time out of mind, the origin of which no one knows. Concerning its meaning there has been. prodigious dispute. It is sufficient to say that it has puzzled all the antiquaries in England, to judge from the Transactions of all the learned societies, and reiterated inquiries and examination in *Notes and Queries*, and other professedly explaining periodicals. The supposed aggrieved person, in regard of this singular calling upon the name of Haro, has the right to go into the highway, and to make public protestation of his wrong. He acclaims upon this mysterious name, shouting as if to an imaginary person. He kneels down in the middle of the road, turns his face to the east, like a Mahommedan, raises his voice, and calls aloud upon an invisible somebody, to whom he appeals by the unintelligible name of Haro, Haro, "to the rescue;" invoking help, or a champion, which, in some sort of superstitious, supernatural fashion, the suppliant is imagined thereby to obtain.

That Hercules and his followers of the Phallic sect were driven from Mycenæ by conquerors of the opposite religious party, we deduce from the ruins themselves of the Cyclopæan pyramidal gate of Mycenæ (of which so many puerile and flimsy explanations have been given), whose stupendous triangular pediment, and other appropriate architectural arrangements, prove it to have been constructed by the upholders of a contrary faith. In confirmation of this, we read (vol. v., p. 270, *Asiatic Researches,*) that Diodorus Siculus says, "the posterity of Hercules reigned for many centuries in Pali-bothra (or Baali-putra)," which means literally a country peopled by the children of the sun.

We have here to explain that all Architecture, ancient and modern, is governed simply by two ideas of expression, both of which are eminently Phallic, and full of meaning, certainly of sacred meaning. The governing line of all the temples in the old religions is horizontal; thus the Jewish temple, or tabernacle, line is horizontal, following the form of the ark (*argha, arc, arche,* case or container), the oblong magical depository of the mysteries, in the *penetralia* of which, the altar-fire, or fire of the gods, is to burn. This is the shrine of the gods, the container of gods or their images. The Egyptian temples—the architectural wonders of the world—are vast, horizontal, hieroglyphic-covered bulks, severe, ponderous, pyramidal, impressive only of gloom, and of majestic, though terrible rites always. The Greek temples, with their elaborate, richly-detailed friezes, resembled long chests, with rows of colonnades stretching down the sides, and widened on platforms, or *stylobates,* as they are technically called. Besides, following out the same levelled lines, which expressed the architectural feminine idea, there were the magnificent depressed pediments, the *tympana* of which were filled with mythological sculpture. These were the *tetrastyles, sestyles, octostyles, decastyles,* or *dodecastyles,* into which the grades of the frontal and rearward colonnades of the temples were distinguished; the *porticus pronaos,* and *posticus,* were technical names of the grand colonnades east and west.

Over all, the glory of the sun of the Olympian
. Greece was lavished. All the temples, and their majestic
detail, were made up to the sight in the superb, deeply-
sunk, architectural shadows, the grandeur and the beauty
of which are known only to the artist, revelling as he .
does upon the pictorial wonders of Grecian colonnades,
entablatures, pediment, *lacunæ* (in the interiors), and
mouldings, and the outlines that exhaust elegance and
taste, literally.

The Roman temples indicate the same feminine lateral
line and horizontal extension. This horizontal architectural form was that sacred to the feminine mysticism.
Construction of this character hinted the adoption of the
female idea, as to the principal ruling power. But the
ascending or aspiring line, such as that of the perpendicular Phallus, or obelisk, meant the opposite idea, or
the male influence. This was the Phallus or Phallos
(φαλλος), proper, the masculine upright, the ascending,
forceful assertion of armed nature, the column of slender,
sworded, celestial Fire.

The double *Lithoi*, or Phalli, are twin powers, or
double, just as Light itself is a twin power, or double, in
its own nature and capacity, for it is not only light, but
also, and at the same time, the Matter out of which light
is made; the light being always the brighter, in proportion as the substantive matter which supplies its life
(magically), is the thickest and the densest. All this is
well understood among the most acute and the soundest
naturalists and physiologists. These are the gods of the
Phalli; for, in the philosophic, theosophic, theogonic
sense, the Phalli are not idols. They are Male-Female,
Mind-Matter, Sun-Moon, Heaven-Earth, Conception-

Image, Fire-Water; the Upright Line and the Lateral Line together constituting the Cross, and (farther) the cross of Crucifixion. Which of all this—Two Senses, or Double Sense, or United Sense in Double Sense—which of all is first? or which *can* be first in dignity, when we examine abstractions so profound, and so evading, and metaphysics so extremely attenuated and shadowy?

We may now pass on to the results of these curious inquiries as to the real meaning of the Phalli, the overpowering significance of which has been too much ignored. The Phalli are sacred monuments, but, for fear of certain ideas that might be raised in relation to them, many worthy scholars shrink from them. We aim in our dissertation, involving the architectural and archæological points of our general subject, at explaining the value of a system of interpretation which seems to contain the only key for expounding the religious mysteries of all nations, or which may prevail to open the sealed historic volume that contains the records of long bygone antiquity, and a whole round of interesting puzzles. The riches obtainable in the more remote and hidden departments of this Phallic, and consequently Gnostic, subject, we may almost say are inexhaustible. We have carefully refrained from straying in, or have only discursively visited, those tempting nooks and avenues, those inviting paths whose bright vistas, branching out of the subject, would have led us undesirably far. But keeping the straight line traced out for our purpose, we find ourselves, as it were, arrived at the shores of an ocean which abounds indeed in precious spoils, but which time will not admit the means of adequately securing. However, we seek, in all proper, justifiable respects, to

fathom a doctrine which, more than any other ever
broached, promises to unravel and disentangle the real
history of mankind, the true causes of their ancient wars
and emigrations, and of their institutions from the earliest
records of humanity, and which *certainly affords the only
rational clue to the mazes of universal mythology.*

Sir William Jones has casually remarked on the
analogy between the Gothic, Celtic, and Persian, with
the Sanscrit; on the identity of many of the Indian,
Egyptian, and Grecian gods; on the analogy between
Peru and part of India; on the early connexion between
India and Africa; on the probability of Ireland being
peopled by Persian migration. But if the foregoing
principles that guided that process of inquiry by which
we clearly identified the worship of the Mexicans and of
the ancient Chinese (by an inquisition into the radical
names and natures of their temples and their gods) were
followed up and duly carried out by men of real erudition,
conversant with primitive and radical languages, and
ancient universal history, we are persuaded that—by a
strict etymological inquiry into the *proper names* (with
all their ramifications) of the countries, of the gods, and
of the temples of the ancients, in connexion with the
foregoing theories—we might arrive at a knowledge
of the universal history of the world, far exceeding in
scientific interest any yet possessed, and at a complete
and satisfactory elucidation of innumerable obscure and
enigmatical facts relative to the vestiges and records
which remain of the nations of old, whether architectural,
mythological, or historical, and which only afford food for,
we had almost said, irrational conjecture, vague surmise,
or puerile and pedantic disquisition.

Very recently a most industrious author and antiquary, who spent many years on military service in India, laboriously and enthusiastically, recognising the importance of his quest into the meaning of worships, made comparison of the monuments, to deduce the tokens of real religion. He found them all, on close and critical examination, to mean but the one thing, the very Phallic worship which in remote days overspread the whole world, and which has left its living remains, even conspicuously to be observed about us *in our own day*, with solid foundations actually in our own religion, and in every intelligible form of Christianity.

Major-General Forlong's book, entitled " The Rivers of Life: An Account of the Faiths,"—abounding in illustrations, and published in two elaborate quarto volumes,—is to a very considerable extent Godfrey Higgins over again. And Godfrey Higgins' encyclopædic works may be considered as seriously compromising, nay as destructive of, real lively faith and real religion; because that which is supernatural is submitted to realistic questioning that damages the mystery in which yet truly lies the power and the force of all religions. We however repudiate in this present book all idea of offering to the reader anything but " construction;" true, although doubtless it will prove to be profound, mystical, strictly " Christian" paradoxical construction. We contend for *special revelation*, necessarily wrapt up in mysteries. We maintain the *possibility of miracle* in the mysteries of God; although in the world, and in the ideas of the world, there is nothing more fixed and true than the impossibility of miracle. The principle for which we contend throughout all our statements and arguments is that the ideas of man—such a limited, vain creature as he is, beside the Mighty Powers outside of him—are all wrong and absurd, and that his common sense and his ' reason' are utterly no reason at all. These ambitious* attempts to wrestle with Divinity—not in the mystic senses involved in the matching of his powers with the Angel of the Lord, in the figurative struggle of the Patriarch, when on his journey, in the emblematic Scriptures, he meets and strives with the Mysterious Being sent on a message to him—are but the puffed-up vanity, as it were, of the *over-educated*, audacious *child!*

We are all for *construction*—even for *Christian*, although, of course, philosophical, *construction*. We have nothing to do with reality, in man's limited, mechanical, scientific sense, or with *realism*. We have undertaken to show that mysticism is the very life and soul of

---

* Let the words of Goethe always be present to men gifted with habits of thought, if they, at the same time, happen to be blest with penetration.—" The marionette fable of Faust," says Goethe, " murmured with many voices in my soul. I too had wandered into every department of knowledge, and had returned early enough satisfied with the vanity of science. And life, too, I had tried under various aspects, and always came back sorrowing and unsatisfied."

Let such seeker check himself, and recur to the wise warnings supplied poetically in Christopher Marlowe's " Faustus"—the unquestionable original of all the " Fausts," and their instigator—these subjects of the daring man, and the too ambitious and questioning and defiant *learned* man, inducing him to overpass his nature, and to "rush in"—like the fool—where " Angels fear to tread."

> "Cut is the branch that might have grown full straight,
>   And burned is Apollo's laurel-bough,
>   That sometime grew within this learned man ;
>   Whose fiendful fortune may exhort the wise
>   Only to wonder at unlawful things,
>   Whose deepness doth entice such forward wits."

religion; that rites and ritual and formal worship and
prayers are of the absolute necessity of things; that *the
Bible is only misread and misrepresented when rejected as
advancing supposed fabulous and contradictory things;*
that Moses did not make mistakes, but spoke to the
" children of men" in the only way in which *children,* in
their nonage, can be addressed;—that the world is,
indeed, a very different place from that which it is assumed
to be; that what is derided as superstition is the only
true and the only scientific *knowledge;* and, moreover,
that modern knowledge, and modern science, are to a great
extent not only *superstition,* but superstition of a very
destructive and deadly kind.

In the first book which we published concerning these
subjects, and in beginning our design to bring to the contemporaneous knowledge some true ideas of the ROSI-
CRUCIANS, we descanted in a work* called " The Indian
Religions; or Results of the Mysterious Buddhism," on the
fact of Stonehenge being phallic in its design and purpose,
a phallic temple of an antiquity prodigious, even probably
a relic of the First Dispersion; and we stated that it
expressed deified phallicism in perplexing but convincing
forms all over it. Such statements were, of course, greatly
to the consternation of jog-trot believers, who could not,
for a moment, conceive that such extraordinary, and supposedly *indecent,* things were possible. Doubtless, at

---

* " London Asiatic Society.—' The subject of Rāmā, or Boodh,
and the Buddhists, or Bhuddists, is so enveloped in obscurity, but still
of such deep interest, that it is well worthy the attention of the learned
and curious; for it is a religion that has spread far and wide; of which
Fo in China was the chief; and which it is said *is recognised in this
country,* at *Stonehenge.'* " " The Wonders of Elora; or The Narrative
of a Journey in India." By JOHN B. SEELY, Captain B.N.I. London:
1825. See also Godfrey Higgins' " Anacalypsis," " Celtic Druids," &c.

first, the safely-moving, would-be respectable antiquarian world, and, still more suspiciously, the rigidly judicious Christian and the orthodox, were full of disbelief and disapproval. Yet they are, now, fast changing their opinions, and giving in one after the other, more or less reluctantly, in the face of such insurmountable evidence. But, as yet, they do not fully see the majesty and grandeur, and even the profoundly sublime, Christian beautiful side in the mysterious and solemn sense of this truly great subject; so guardedly watched by the philosophers and mystics of all time.

We find that Major-General Forlong has adopted all our references, made so long ago, as to the sexual meanings of the myth indicated in Stonehenge. He treats of it as a Phallic monument, and places his mysterious "Snake," whose effigy is the key and symbol of all these Lunar Theosophic reveries, immediately in front of and below his drawing of Stonehenge. He identifies the symbol with the singular object, standing solitarily in advance of Stonehenge, popularly known under the name of the "Friar's Heel."* This upright, dark stone, which rears itself singularly and weirdly in the solitude, and stands by itself, some distance in advance of the circles of gigantic *Trilithoi*, collectively called "Stonehenge," is strangely changed in its transmission down to modern times, and is now passed off into a masquerade of

* The "Friar's Heel," always anxiously shown to every visitor and explorer at Stonehenge, is a dark, formless, oblong stone, evidently in direct connexion with, but placed much in advance of, the grand exterior circle of stones. It is the same kind of stone, and of about the same significance, as the famous Cab, Keb, Kebla, or Caaba; or Beth-el, Bothel, or "House of God"—or central-point for adoration for the *Hadgis*, or pilgrims to the sacred Mecca,—which is, as is well known, the "Jerusalem" of the Mahommedans.

lingual transformation or re-rendering. This commemorative stone, or upright, is no "Friar's Heel," as it is familiarly designated; but it is a Lingham or Phallus, and is dedicated to Freya or Freia, or the "Friday Divinity," god or goddess, for there is no sex in these respects; it is either or both, as an abstraction or a personified Idea. It is a Friday god or goddess, or a queen, Venus or Aphrodite, Bhaga, or the "Genius of Fire," not, of course, the genius of ordinary fire, but of the supersensual, superessential, divinely operative, celestial Fire.

Obelisks have been raised as sacred mystical objects, and bowed before as idols in all ages; looked upon, mystically and figuratively, as the "Keys of Paradise." We in England should properly have set our greatest archæological acquisition, the Obelisk, not as at present, standing in its mistaken, mean position, amidst the angles of the Thames Embankment; but, imitating the ancients, and the acute, judicious, artistic people of the middle ages, in Italy and elsewhere, we should have placed this priceless, magnificent Memphian trophy between Sir Christopher Wren's kingly towers, flanking the western porticoes of Saint Paul's Cathedral; and having raised this magic Emperor of the Uprights in front of our colossal Christian Temple, we should have crowned and surmounted him with the glorious symbol of the "Saviour" (in this Christian country), emphasising and capping the splendours and dignities of all the gods of all the thousands of years of Egypt, with the triumphant Cross! Such would, indeed, have been a worthy object for the multitude of London to gaze at. But London is confessedly not Athens, any more than any one of its metropolitan and corporate administrators has ever proved himself a Phidias, or a Pericles.

CHAPTER IV.

CELESTIAL, OR THEOSOPHICAL DOCTRINE OF THE UNSEXUAL,
TRANSCENDENTAL PHALLICISM.

OVER the porticoes of all the Egyptian temples, the
winged disc of the sun is placed between two hooded
snakes (the *cobra capello*), signifying that luminary placed
between its two great attributes of motion and life. The
same combination of symbols, to express the same attributes, is observable upon the coins of the Phœnicians
and Carthaginians. (*Médailles de Dutens*, p. 1 ; *Mus.
Hunter*, tab. 15, fig. 5, and viii.) These same symbols
also appear to have been anciently employed by the
Druids of Britain and Gaul, as they still are by the
idolaters of China. See Stukeley's *Abury;* the original
name of which temple, he observes, was the "Snake's
Head :" and it is remarkable that the remains of a
similar circle of stones in Bœotia had the same name in
the time of Pausanias. The Scandinavian goddess, Isa or
Disa, was sometimes represented between two serpents
[*Ol. Rudbeck Atlant.*, pt. iii., c. 1, p. 25, and pt. ii.,
p. 343, fig. A, and p. 510]; and a similar mode of
canonisation is employed in the apotheosis of Cleopatra,
as expressed on her coins.

Perpetual lamps are kept burning in the inmost recesses
of all the great pagodas in India, the Hindoos holding
Fire to be the essence of all active power in nature.
Numa is said to have consecrated the perpetual Fire, as
the first of all things, and the soul of matter; which

without it, is motionless and dead. Fires of the same kind
were, for the same reasons, preserved in most of the
principal temples, both Greek and Barbarian; there being
scarcely a country in the world where some traces of the
adoration paid to fire are not to be found. [*Huet. De-
monst. Evang. Præp.*, iv., c. 5; *Lafitau, Mœurs*, t. i.,
p. 153.] The *prytanæa* of the Greek cities are the points
where the sacred fires were burned in the Temples.

The characteristic attribute of the passive generative
power was expressed in symbolical writing by different
enigmatical representations of the most distinctive characteristic of the sex; such as the Shell, called the
Concha Veneris [*August. de Civ. Dei*, lib. vi., c. 9], the Fig-
leaf [*Plutarch de Is. et Osir*, p. 365], the Barley-corn
[*Eustath. in Homer*, p. 134], or the letter *Delta* [*Suidas*];
all of which occur very frequently upon coins and other
ancient monuments, in this sense. The same attribute,
personified as the goddess of love or desire, is usually
represented under the voluptuous form of a beautiful
naked woman, frequently distinguished by one of these
symbols, and called Venus, Cypris, or Aphroditè, names
of rather uncertain etymology. Other attributes of the
goddess of beauty were on some occasions added, whence
the symbolical statue of Venus at Paphos had a beard,
and other appearances of virility; which seems to have
been the most ancient mode of representing the celestial,
as distinguished from the popular, goddess of that name;
the one being a personification of a general procreative
power, and the other only of animal desire. [*Signum et
hujus Veneris est Cypri barbatum corpore, sed veste muliebri,
cum sceptro et statura viri. Macrob.*, lib. iii., p. 74.] The
fig was a still more common symbol; the statues of Priapus

being made of the tree, and the fruit being carried with the *phallus* in the ancient processions in honour of Bacchus. Whence we often see portraits of persons in Italy painted with the fig in one hand, to signify their orthodox devotion to the fair sex. [See portrait of Tassoni prefixed to the 4to edition of the *Secchia Rapita*, &c.] Hence, also, arose the Italian expression "*far-la-fica;*" which was done by putting the thumb between the middle and forefingers, as it appears in many Priapic ornaments now extant; or by putting the finger or the thumb into the corner of the mouth, and drawing it down; of which there is a representation in a small Priapic figure of exquisite sculpture engraved among the Antiquities of Herculanæum. (*Bronzi.*, tab. xciv.)

It is to these obscene gestures that the expressions of "figging," and "biting the thumb," which Shakespeare probably took from translations of Italian novels, seem to allude. [See 1 *Henry IV.*, Act V., sc. 3, and *Romeo and Juliet*, Act I., sc. 1.] Another old writer, who probably understood Italian, calls the latter "giving the fico;" and, according to its ancient meaning, it might very naturally be employed as a silent reproach of effeminacy.

The key, which is still worn, with the Priapic hand, as an amulet, by the women of Italy, appears to have been an emblem of similar meaning, as the equivocal use of the name of it, in the language of that country, implies. Of the same kind, too, appears to have been the cross in the form of the letter T, attached to a circle, which all, or most, of the figures of Egyptian deities, both male and female, carry in the left hand, and by which the Syrians, Phœnicians, and other inhabitants of Asia, represented the planet Venus—worshipped by them as the natural emblem or image of that goddess. [*Procli. Paraphr.*, lib. ii., p. 97. See also *Mich. Ang.* " *De la chausse*," part ii., No. xxxvi., fol. 62, and *Jablonski Panth.*, *Egypt.*, lib. ii., c. vii., s. 6.] The cross in this form is sometimes observable on coins; and several of them were found in a temple of Serapis, demolished at the general destruction of those edifices by the emperor Theodosius; and were said, by the Christian antiquaries of that time, to signify the future life. [*Suidas in v.,* ταυρος.] In solemn sacrifices all the Lapland idols were marked with it from the blood of the victims [*Scheffer, Lappanic,* c. x., p. 112]; and it occurs on many Runic monuments found in Sweden and Denmark, which are of an age long anterior to the approach of Christianity to those countries; and, probably, to its appearance in the world. [*Ol. Rudbeck, Atlant.*, p. ii., c. xi., p. 662, and p. 111, c. i., s. iii.; *Ol. Varelli Scandagr. Runic; Borlase, Hist. of Cornwall*, p. 106.] On some of the early coins of the Phœnicians, we find it attached to a chaplet of beads placed in a circle, so as to form a complete rosary. From the very name of "rosary," in connexion with these ultra-remote matters, we can perceive the *replication*—if we may make use of such a word—of the Rosicrucian adepts to these far-off and figurative views of the mysterious relationship of the Cross and Rose: and, moreover, of the meanings conveyed through the apocalyptic symbol of the "Crucified-Rose;" which, to ordinary understandings, is unintelligible, and a masquerade—although a signally grand, significant " masquerade"—only to be played before and presented to the apprehension of the true Rosicrucian Initiates. The " Rosary," as a form, is precisely the same symbol, although the devotees are mainly, if not wholly, in a state of ignorance as to the real meanings conveyed in all the ideas which go with it; the same in the hands, and in the use, of the Lamas of Thibet and China, the Hindoos, the more profound sects among the Buddhists, and the Roman Catholics—at least among the most deeply-thinking and penetrating of them. [*Pellerin, Villes.*, t. ii., pl. cxxii., fig. 4; *Archæol.*, vol. xiv., p. 2; *Nichoff.*, s. ix.; *Maurice, Indian Antiquities*, vol. v.]

The Scandinavian goddess, Freya, had (like the Paphian Venus) the characteristics of both sexes. [*Mallet Hist. de Danemarc, Introd.*, c. vii., p. 116.]

Considering the general state of reserve and restraint in which the Grecian women lived, it is astonishing to what an excess of extravagance their religious enthusiasm was carried on certain occasions; particularly in celebrating the orgies of Bacchus. The gravest matrons and proudest princesses suddenly laid aside their decency and their dignity, and ran screaming among the woods and mountains, fantastically dressed or half naked, with hair dishevelled and interwoven with ivy or vine, and sometimes with living serpents. [*Plutarch in Alexandr.*] In this manner they frequently worked themselves up to such a pitch of savage ferocity, as not only to feed upon raw flesh (*Apollon. Rhod.*, lib. i., 636, and *Schol.*), but even to tear living animals to pieces with their teeth, and eat them warm and palpitating. [*Jul. Firmic.*, c. 14; *Clement. Alex. Cohort.*, p. ii.; *Arnob.*, lib. v.] The enthusiasm of the Greeks was, however, generally of the gay and festive kind; which almost all their religious rites tended to promote. Music and wine always accompanied devotion, as tending to exhilarate men's minds, and assimilate them with the deity; to imitate whom was to feast and rejoice, to cultivate the elegant and useful arts ; and thereby to give and receive happiness (*Strabo*, lib. x., p. 476).

The Babylonian women of every rank and condition held it to be an indispensable duty of religion to prostitute themselves, once in their lives, in the temple of Mylitta, who was the same goddess as the Venus of the Greeks, to any stranger who came and offered money; which, whether little or much, was accepted, and applied to sacred purposes. Numbers of these devout ladies were always in waiting, and the stranger had the liberty, regulated by a certain determining form of lot, of choosing in whatever direction his liking should prevail, as the women reclined in rows in the walks about the temple, guarded by the sacred usages, but exposed otherwise freely enough; no refusal being allowed (*Herodotus*, lib. i.). A similar custom prevailed in Cyprus (*Herod.*, c. 199), and probably in many other countries, it being, as Herodotus observes, the practice of all mankind, except the Greeks and Egyptians, to take such liberties with their temples, which, they concluded, must be pleasing to the Deity, since birds and animals, acting under the guidance of instinct, or by the immediate impulse of Heaven, did the same. The exceptions he might safely have omitted, at least so far as relates to the Greeks; for there were a thousand sacred prostitutes kept in each of the celebrated temples of Venus, at Eryx and Corinth; who, according to all accounts, were extremely expert and assiduous in attending to the duties of their profession. (*Strabo*, lib. viii.; *Diodor. Sic.*, lib. iv.; *Philodemi Epigr. in Brunck. Analect.*, vol. ii., p. 85.) It is not likely that the temple which they served should be the only place exempt from being the scene of these freedoms. Dionysius of Halicarnassus claims the same exception in favour of the Romans, but, as we suspect, equally without reason; for Juvenal, who lived only a century later, when the same religion and nearly the same manners prevailed, seems to consider every temple in Rome as a kind of licensed brothel :—

> " Nuper enim, ut repeto, fanum Isidis et Ganymeden,
> Pacis, et advectæ secreta palatia matris,
> Et Cererem, (nam quo non prostat femina templo?)
> Notior Aufidis mæchas celebrare solebas."—*Sat.* ix., 22.

While the temples of the Hindoos possessed their establishments, most of them had bands of consecrated prostitutes, called the Women of the Idol, selected in their infancy by the Brahmins for the beauty of their persons, and trained up with every elegant accomplishment that could render them attractive, and insure success in the profession which they exercised at once for the pleasure and profit of the priesthood.   They were never allowed to desert the temple; and the offspring of their promiscuous embraces were, if males, consecrated to the service of the deity in the ceremonies of his worship; and, if females, educated in the profession of their mothers.   (*Maurice Antiq. Ind.*, vol. i., part i., p. 341.)

Night, being the appropriate season for these mysteries, and being also supposed to have some genial and nutritive influence in itself (*Orph. Hymn.* ii. 2), was personified as the source of all things, the passive productive principle of the universe (*Diodor. Sic.*, I., i., c. vii.), which the Egyptians called by a name that signified "night"— Αθυρ or Αθωρ, *called Athorh still in the Coptic.* (*Jablonski, Panth. Egypt.*, lib. i., c. i., s. 7.)   Hesiod says that "the nights belong to the blessed gods; as it is then that dreams descend from Heaven to forewarn and instruct

men." (*Hesiod.* Ερy. 730.) Hence Night is called
ευφρονη, *good,* or *benevolent,* by the ancient poets; and to
perform any unseemly act or gesture in the face of night,
(though still more in the face of the sun) was accounted
a heinous offence. (*Hesiod.* Ερy. 727.) This may seem,
indeed, a contradiction to their practice: but it must be
remembered that a free communication between the sexes
was never reckoned criminal by the ancients, unless when
injurious to the peace or pride of families; and as to the
foul and unnatural debaucheries imputed to the Baccha-
nalian societies suppressed by the Romans, they were either
mere calumnies, or abuses introduced by private persons,
and never countenanced by public authority in any part
of the world. Had the Christian societies sunk under
the first storms of persecution, posterity might have
believed them guilty of similar crimes; of which they
were equally accused by witnesses as numerous. (*Liv.
Hist.,* l. xxxix., c. 9, &c. *Mosheim,* &c.) We do,
indeed, sometimes find indications of unnatural lusts in
ancient sculptures: but " they were undoubtedly the works
of private caprice; or similar compositions would have
been found upon coins; which they never are, except
upon the 'Spintriæ' of Tiberius, which are supposed
to have been merely tickets of admission to the scenes of
his private amusement. Such preposterous appetites,
though but too observable in all the later ages of Greece,
appear to have been wholly unknown to the simplicity of
the early times; they never being once noticed either in
the Iliad, the Odyssey, or the genuine poem of Hesiod;
for as to the lines in the former poem alluding to the
rape of Ganymede, they are manifestly spurious." (*Il.
E.,* 265, &c. Y. 230, &c.)

This may be very true to a certain extent. But unfortunately, from the testimony of all antiquity—and certainly modern readers endeavour to think the best of the ancient times—we are compelled to believe that the sins and enormities of the early generations were awful indeed. We encounter enough of all this "ruinous side of human life" in the Scriptures, and gather accounts of it from the earliest historians, who, in their general taste, perhaps, also, from fear, seem desirous of not saying too much. There is reason to believe that the world before the Deluge—of which "Deluge," even in its *total* character, there is more than enough proof in the accounts of all the nations, in the penetrative critical mind—was filled with monstrous sins and wickedness, and crimes against nature itself—even *scientific* man being degraded worse than the brutes.

CHAPTER V.

THE MYSTERIES OF THE PHALLUS. ITS IDEALISED GNOSTIC,
ROSICRUCIAN, OR CHRISTIAN RENDERINGS.

THOUGH the Greek writers call the deity who was represented by the sacred goat at Mendes, Pan, he more exactly answers to Priapus, or the generative attribute considered abstractedly (*Diodor. Sic.*, lib. i., p. 78); which was usually represented in Egypt, as well as in Greece, by the Phallus only. (*Ibid.*, p. 16.) This deity was honoured with a place in most of their temples (*Ibid.*), as the Lingam, or Lingham, is in those of the Hindoos; and all the hereditary priests were initiated or consecrated to him, before they assumed the sacerdotal office (*Ibid.*, p. 78): he was considered as a sort of accessory attribute to all the other divine personifications; and truly so, for without this, or some similar means or machinery, they themselves obviously could not be. The very root and foundation of the Buddhistic theosophical ideas is the impossibility of any phases or forms of being, or recognition, existing otherwise than as evil. All the mistakes of theologians are derived from their reluctance to admit the idea that *Nirwan*, or *Nirwana*, of the Buddhists means annihilation, or absorption into nothing, which, in truth, the real Buddhism teaches. But this *substratum*, or ground principle of Buddhism, "annihilation," is not to be taken in the way which these erroneous construers of Buddhism suppose. The broad outline of the Buddhist philosophy is a proposition, that all comprehensible existence, that all forms, phases, or formularies of existence, all emotion of any kind, stir, or sense of individuality—the *cogito, ergo sum*, of Descartes; that everything, in fact, is only good or bad relatively; that in reality, apart from manifestation or acceptance of the thing, there is *nothing either good or evil;* being only good or evil in man's necessitated self-delusion: that all life, particularly human life, is a parade of *phenomena,* of whatever character the movement operating may be. It will follow, conclusively, that extrication, rescue, or permanent and perfect deliverance out of this Masquerade of Being, totally different to what it seems, is Heaven; and that this state of bliss is attainable by the perfect Bhuddists, in withdrawing out of being by repeated purifications, assisted by the multitudinous spirits, into that *Nirvana* which these abstruse fantastic religionists deem the blessed state of ultimate, never-ending rhapsody of perfect quiet, clear of all stimulus of consciousness. This is an ecstatic state, impossible of deviation, or change. It is the last Light, the *Pleroma,* or fulness of everything. It may, doubtless, be true, that the philosophy of Buddhism is a shadowy philosophy; but this is the true intent and purpose of it; and, we think, just as clearly stated.

Amidst the Phallic ideas, the prevailing persuasion is that all the divine personifications imply that their great end and purpose—and the very explanation and justification of their existence—is generation, production, or renovation; general replacement, in fact. A part of the worship offered to the goat, Mendes, and the bull, Apis, consisted in the women tendering to him their persons, which it seems the former often accepted, though the taste of the latter was too correct. (*Pindar. apud Strabon.*, xvii., p. 802 ; *Herodot.*, lib. ii., s. 46 ; *Diodor. Sic.*, lib. i.) An attempt seems to have been made, in early times, to introduce similar acts of devotion into Italy ; for when the oracle of Juno was consulted upon the long-continued barrenness of the Roman matrons, its answer was, " Iliadas matres caper hirtus inito ;" but these mystic refinements not being understood by this *unintelligent* people, they could think of no other interpretation, and truly of no other way of fulfilling the mandate, than sacrificing a goat, and applying the skin, cut into thongs, to the bare backs of the ladies—*whipping them, in fact.* This is the origin of a certain kind of flagellation. " Jussæ sua terga maritæ pellibus exsectis percutienda dabant ;" which, however, had the desired effect, " Virque pater subito, nuptaque mater erat." (*Ovid. Fast.*, ii., 448.)

This explains the flogging of the women at the ceremonies of the Lupercal at Rome, and the directions of Cæsar to his wife Calphurnia, "Stand you directly in Antonius' way when he doth run his course." See Shakespeare's *Julius Cæsar*, in the scene where the Roman games—which, in their mysteries, were all Phallic and astronomical—are referred to. At Mendes, female goats were also held sacred, as symbols of the passive generative attribute (*Strabon.*, lib. xvii., 812) ; and on Grecian monuments of art we often find caprine satyrs of the female sex. A female Pantheic figure in silver, of which an engraving was published by Count Caylus (tome vii., pl. lxxi.), represents Cybele, the universal mother, as mixing the productive elements of heat and moisture— Fire and Water, the two grand components (indicating halves) of the visible world, according to the Rosicrucians—by making a libation upon the flames of an altar from a golden *patera*, with the usual knob in the centre of it, representing, probably, the lingam, and very similar, indeed, to the Indian forms of the same superlative object.

The Disa or Isa of the north was represented by a conic figure. This goddess is delineated on the sacred drums of the Laplanders as accompanied by a child, similar to the Horus of the Egyptians, who so often appears in the lap of Isis, on the religious monuments of that people. (*Isiac Table, and Ol. Rudbeck. Atlant.*, pp. 209 and 210; *Ib.*, p. 280.)

The ancient Muscovites also worshipped a similar sacred group, probably representing Isis and her offspring. They had likewise another idol, called the golden heifer, which seems to have been the animal symbol of the same personage.

The conic form unquestionably means the egg; the top, or culminating part of the Phallus. Thus it stands in all minarets, or circular towers. The piercing point of the *gladius* is also indubitably marked out in the summit part of all the obelisks. The origin of which word, *Obelisc*, we may here notice, has been demonstrated as coming from two Hebrew or Chaldaic terms, *ob*, meaning " snake," " serpent," " *magic*," and *lis*, or *lisc*, signifying, in certain mythic inflections, " Fire." *Obelos*, in the Greek, is also a " spit, brand, or dart" as the rays of the sun, the active, motived " fire," are darted.

The ancient nations of the north consecrated each day of the week to some principal personage of their mythology, and called it after his name, beginning with Lok or Saturn, and ending with Freia or Freya, the Scandinavian Venus, or the Genius of the "Fateful Friday," a day of days in the "left-handed" superstitions of all countries.

Of monumental stones of a conical form, the Phallic or Priapic type has especially at all periods been *human*, from the crown of the head to the line of the ventral region, or the line of the double division, taking start at the centre point between the thighs. This significant, mathematical, also mystical form is represented upon the colonial medals of Tyre by monuments of conic shape called "ambrosial" stones; from which, probably, came the amberics, so frequent all over the northern hemisphere. These, from the remains still extant, appear to have been composed of one of these cones let into the ground, with another stone placed upon the point of it (Bowing-Stones), and so nicely balanced that the wind could move it, though so ponderous that no human force, unaided by machinery, can displace it. Whence they are also called "Logging-Rocks," and Pender or Pendre-Stones (Norden's *Cornwall*, p. 79), as they were anciently "Living-Stones," and "Stones of God" (*Pseudo-Sanchon. Fragm. apud Euseb.* "βαιτυλια."). The last title seems to be a corruption of the scriptural name, "Bethel." In truth, it is the same thing.

Damascius saw several of these stones in the neighbourhood of Heliopolis or Baalbeck, in Syria; and mentions one which was then moved by the wind (*In vitâ Isidori apud Phot. Biblioth. Cod.* 242). These oracular stones, or speaking Idols (for such all these monuments are), are equally found in the western extremities of Europe and the eastern extremities of Asia; in Britain, notably at Stonehenge, which is a temple of these idols, and at Abury, or Avebury, which is a temple of mystical stones dedicated to the worship of the Serpent. From the westernmost limit of Europe (at the margin of the Atlantic, at Carnac, in Brittany,) to the easternmost frontier of China, these supposed "enchanted stones" are to be found—stone letters (or "tabulates" inscribed), scattered broadcast, of the original faith—the signals and hieroglyphics of which seem to have been dropped at the beginning of historical time from heaven, each stone stored, it may be said, invisibly with the original Promethean fire.

CHAPTER VI.

RITES AND CEREMONIES OF THE INDIAN PHALLIC WORSHIP, AND ITS CONNEXION WITH GENERAL RELIGIOUS MEANINGS.

DANCING formed an important part of the ceremonial worship of most Eastern peoples. Dancing girls were attached to the Egyptian and also to the Jewish temples. David, also, as we are told, "danced before the Lord with all his might." And to every temple of any importance, in India, we find a *Nautch*, or troop of dancing girls attached. These women are generally procured when quite young, and are early initiated into all the mysteries of the profession. They are instructed in dancing, and vocal and instrumental music, their chief employment being to chant the sacred hymns, and perform *nautches* before the god, on the recurrence of high festivals. But this is not the only, and, in peculiar senses, not the most important, and certainly not the most seductive service required of them; for besides being the acknowledged mistresses of the officiating priests, it is their duty to prostitute themselves, in the courts of the temples, to all comers, and thus raise funds for the enrichment of the place of worship to which they belong.

They are always women of considerable personal attractions, and sometimes boasting the most remarkable beauty, either of face or form, and very frequently of both combined. These special allurements of countenance and shape are heightened by all the choice blandishments of dress, manner of disposal of dress (or undress), jewels, accomplishments, and art; so that they frequently receive large sums in return for the favours they grant, and fifty, one hundred, and even two hundred rupees have been known to be paid to these syrens for one night's possession.

Nor are these usages very much to be wondered at, as these females comprise among their number perhaps some of the loveliest women in the world. All temptations are heightened by their secrecy, and by their being artfully kept back.

It has been said already, that among the classes from which a medium for *sacti* is selected, is the courtesan and dancing-girl grade. They are, indeed, more frequently chosen for this honour than others. A *Nautch* woman esteems it a peculiar privilege to become *Radha Dea* on such occasions. It is an office the duties of which these adepts are, on every account, better calculated to fulfil with satisfaction to the sect of *Sacteyas* who may require their aid, than a more innocent and unsophisticated girl.

The worship of *Sacti* is the adoration of Power, which the Hindüs typify by the *Yoni*, or womb, the *Argha*, or *vulva*, and by the leaves and flowers of certain plants, thought to resemble it. Thus we find in the *Ananda-Tantram* (c. vi., verse 13) an allusion to the *Aswattha*, or sacred fig-tree, the leaf of which is in the shape of a heart, and much resembles the conventional form of the *yoni*, to which it is compared.

> " Aswattha patrasadrusam Yoniáciáram chabhàjànam.
> Támra, rúpya, suvaruaistu rachitam tal prasasyate."

In Egypt, we learn that *Typho* sometimes bore the name of *Setho*, "by which they mean the 'tyrannical and overbearing Power,' or, as the word frequently signifies, 'the Power that overturns all things, and that overleaps all bounds.'" (*Plutarch, de Iside et Osiride,* xxxvi.)

In *Ananda-Tantram,* cap. vii., 148, and other passages, reference is made to *Bhagamala.* She appears to be the goddess who presides over the *pudendum-muliebre, i.e.* the deified *Vulva;* and the *Sacti* is thus personified. In the mental adoration of Sacti a diagram is framed, and the figure imagined to be seen inside the *Vulva.* This is the *Adhó-mukham,* or lower face, *i.e.* the *Yoni,* wherein the worshipper is to imagine (*mantapam*) a chapel to be erected. (*Ananda-Tantram.*) All the forms of *Sacti-puja* require the use of some or all of the five *Makaras.* They are enumerated in the *Syama Rahasya.* "*Mudra* and Maithuna are the fivefold *Makára,* which take away all sin." The five *Makaras* are *mansa, matsya, madya, maithuna,* and *mudra;* that is flesh, fish, wine, women, and certain mystical twistings or gesticulations with the fingers. Such are some of the peculiar features of the worship of Power (GNOSTICISM), which combined with the Linga-Puja (adoration of the Phallus), constitutes at the present day one of the most popular dogmas of the Hindüs.

Simon Magus is supposed to have been the founder of western Gnosticism. He it was who corrupted the Nicolaitans. (*Vid. Apocalypse,* ii., 6, 15.) They held sensual pleasure to be the true creed. In the *Foreign Quarterly Review* (pp. 159, 160), the following passage occurs :—"The grand object of the magic of the Christians in the middle ages was to obtain the command over the services of demons ; such were the pursuits of witches. But these were always looked upon as criminal. The belief that men possess the power to control spirits was

not peculiar to the Gnostic Christians. The liturgies of
the Roman and Greek Churches contain several rules on
these subjects."

The memoirs of Scipio de Ricci, Bishop of Pistoja,
reveal some remarkable facts, plainly demonstrating that
sacteya ideas had found their way into the monasteries
and convents of Italy in the latter part of the last century.
SELLON does not seem to be aware where Sactinism (or
Sactism) borders on Gnosticism, and where Gnosticism
and Aphroditism pass up into exceptional mysticism; and
again where this latter, which takes in the foundation of
all religion, rises into and evanishes in the irradiation of
Rosicrucianism—last and holiest, and the most abstruse
and abstract of all—spreading and lost in *celestial magic.*
This is the only true faith, because forbidden to all, and
secret to all, in the state of flesh, for Man cannot sustain
the "disclosure of God, and live." Under all this,
Masonry (that is, *authentic* Masonry,) can alone live and
spring.

According to Theodoret, Arnobius, and Clemens of
Alexandria, the *Yoni* of the Hindüs was the sole object
of veneration in the mysteries of Eleusis. (*Demosthenes
on the Crown.*) When the people of Syracuse were
sacrificing to goddesses, they offered cakes in a certain
form, called μυλλοι (*Apuleius*, p. 302); and in some
temples, where the priestesses were probably ventrilo-
quists, they so far imposed on the credulous multitude,
who came to adore the *Vulva,* as to make them believe
that it spoke and gave oracles. The Phallic rites were
so well known among the Greeks that a metre consisting
of three trochees only derived its name therefrom. In the
opinion of those who compiled the *Puranas,* Phallus was

first publicly worshipped by the name of *Básewarra-Linga* on the banks of *Cumudati*, or Euphrates, and the Jews, according to Rabbi Acha, seem to have had some such idea, as may be collected from what is said regarding the different earths which formed the "body of Adam."

In many of the observances practised in the religious solemnities of the Hindoos, solitude is enjoined; but all the principal ceremonies comprehend the worship of *Sacti* or *Power*, and require, for that purpose, the presence of a young and beautiful girl, as the living representative of the goddess. The female, thus worshipped, is ever after denominated *Yogini*, *i.e.* attached. This Sanscrit word is, in the dialects, pronounced *Jogi* or *Zogee*, and is equivalent to a secular *nun*, as these women are subsequently supported by alms. The word, from custom, has become equivalent with *sena*, and thus is exactly the same as *Duti* or *Dutica* (doo-ty-car). The books of morality direct a faithful wife to shun the society of *Yogini*, or females who have been adored as *Sacti*.

The *sacti* system bears a striking affinity with Epicureanism. It teaches materialism, and the Atomic system of chance. (Compare the *Ananda-Tantram*, c. xvii., with *Lucretius*, lib. iii.) The worship of women, and the *Sacta b'oma vidhi*, are grounded on passages in the *Veda* which orthodox Brahmins regard as of doubtful authority. (*Vide Rig. Vedam.*, bk. ii., c. viii., sections 13, 14, 2nd attham, 8th pannam: ricks, b. 14, which contain the "*Sucla Homa Mantram*," &c.)

This worship of the *Sacti* is mostly celebrated in a mixed society, the men of which represent *Bhanravis* and *Nayikas*.

The *Sacti* is personified by a *naked girl*, to whom meat

and wine are offered, and then distributed among the
assistants. Here follows the chanting of the *Muntras*
and sacred Texts, and the performance of the *Mudra*, or
gesticulations with the fingers. The whole terminates
with orgies amongst the votaries of a most licentious
description. (*Wilson on Hin. Sects*, vol. xvii.; *As. Res.
Ward on the Vaisnavas*, p. 309.) This ceremony is
entitled the *Sri Chakra*, or *Purna-bisheka*, the "Ring
or Full Initiation."

This method of adoring the *Sacti* is unquestionably
acknowledged by the Texts, which are regarded by the
Vanis as authorities for the impurities practised. The
members of the sect are sworn to secrecy, and will not
therefore acknowledge any participation in *Sacta-Puja*.
Some years ago, however, they began to throw off this
reserve, and, at the present day, they trouble themselves
very little to disguise their initiation into its mysteries;
but they do not divulge in what those mysteries consist.

The *Culanava* has the following, and other similar
passages; the Tantras also abound with them.

" Many false pretenders to knowledge, and who have
not been duly initiated, pretend to practise the Caula
rites: but if perfection be attained by drinking wine,
then every drunkard is a saint; if virtue consists in eating
flesh, then every carnivorous animal in the world is
virtuous; if eternal happiness be derived from the union
of the sexes, then all beings will be entitled to it. A
follower of the Caula doctrine is blameless in my sight if
he reproves those of other creeds who quit their established observances. Those of other sects who use the
articles of the Caula worship shall be condemned to a
metempsychosis during as many years as there are hairs

of the body." The *Kauchiluas* are another branch of
the Sactas sect; their worship much resembles that of
the Caulas. They are, however, distinguished by one
peculiar rite, not practised by the others, and " throw into
confusion all the ties of female relationship, natural
restraints are wholly disregarded, and a community of
women among the votaries inculcated. On the occasions
of the performance of divine worship, the women and
girls deposit their *Julies*, or bodices, in a box, each
lettered and numbered, in charge of the *Guru*, or priest.
At the close of the rites, the male worshippers take each
a *julie* from the box, and the female to whom the letter
and number appertains, even were she the sister of the
man who draws the lot, is forced, by the inexorable law
of the place, and of the sacred necessities of the service,
to become his conjoint partner for the night in these
lascivious orgies." We are here at once reminded of
the lustful solemnities practised amidst the mysteries of
the temples of the Babylonians; and of the abandonment
to irregular pleasure prevailing in the *penetralia*, where
the rites of the *Bona Dea*, amongst the Romans, were
celebrated by the outwardly accepted chastest, and most
serious and well-mannered women, matrons and girls alike,
of the highest quality in Rome. All these secret festivals or celebrations were sacred, and most carefully
covered, in all their wildest excesses, by the sanctions of
religion, and, incredible as it must appear, all the
solemnities of sacred incidence.

The numerous terra-cotta figures and images in ivory,
to which Layard has given the general name of Venus
(*Kun*), seem unquestionably to be impersonations of
Sacti, or the female power, as the Yoni is rather obtru-

sively represented in many of these statuettes, while the fissure and other natural appendages are absent in others. In the former, not only is the Yoni (or Ioni) portrayed, but "a certain ornament on the *mons veneris* is curled precisely in the same conventional manner as is seen in the beards of the male statues in the Assyrian antiquities. While, in the latter, the true Venus, the fissure, and the appendages are omitted." Why this prudery? The appendages are the surrounding hair.

One is therefore led to believe that the adoration of *Sacti* was a prominent feature in the Assyrian worship. And this idea is confirmed by a *bas-relief* of clay, found at Susa, which gives a nude female, having the *yoni* depicted, and holding in her hands the *Argha* (originals in the British Museum). The attitude of this figure, and the manner in which the *Argha* is placed in her hands, resembles, in a remarkable manner, the images of the Hindu goddess, *Devi*.

CHAPTER VII.

HEBREW PHALLICISM.

In the Gemara Sanhedrim, c. 30, cited by Ryland, will be found many peculiarities of the Hebrew method of dealing with the mystic side of Phallicism.

If reference be made to chap. iv., vol. iii., of Lewis's *Origines Hebraicæ* much curious information will be found regarding the " Idolatry of the Hebrews," which not only plainly shows that they adored Phallus, but goes far to confirm the hypothesis that the object of veneration in the Ark of the Covenant was the emblem itself, or a type of it. At page 23, vol. iii., we read that " the most ancient monuments of idolatry among the Gentiles, were consecrated Pillars (*Lingas ?*) or Columns (Obelisks), which the Hebrews were forbidden to erect as objects of divine homage and adoration." Yet he adds, " This practice is conceived to arise from an *imitation of Jacob*, who took a stone and *set it up*," &c. Again, " This stone was held in great veneration in later times by the Jews and removed to Jerusalem." They were accustomed " to anoint this stone," and from the word " Bethel," " the place where the pillar was erected, came the word Bœtylia among the heathen, which signified rude stones which they worshipped, either as symbols of divinity, or as true gods animated by some heavenly power." Indeed it would seem not improbable that the erection of the *Pillar of Jacob* actually gave rise to the worship of Phallus among some of the pagan peoples. " For," says

Lewis, "the learned Bochart asserts that the Phœnicians, (at least as the Jews think) first worshipped this very stone which Jacob anointed, and afterwards consecrated others," &c. It is to little purpose that we are reminded that the Jews were forbidden by their law to "make unto themselves any graven image," for, as Lewis shows in the following passage, there may be exceptions to this, as to every other general rule :—"Notwithstanding the severity of the law against the making of images, yet, as Justin Martyr observes in his book against Trypho, it must be somewhat mysterious, that God in the case of the Brazen Serpent should command an image to be made ; for which," he says, "one of the Jews confessed he never could hear a reason from any of their doctors."

The Brazen Serpent continued to be worshipped by the Jews, and incense was offered to that idol, till the reign of Hezekiah. "For as it is written in the law of Moses, 'whosoever looks upon it shall live,' they fancied they might obtain blessings by its mediation, and therefore thought it worthy to be worshipped." The learned Dr. Jackson observes, "that the pious Hezekiah was moved with the greater indignation against this image, because in truth it never was a type of our Saviour, but a figure of his grand enemy," &c.

Then we find the Jews- relapsing into idolatry by the adoration of the Golden Calf. In regard to this Golden Calf (which was not a "Golden Calf" at all, but something very different, and of infinitely greater significance), we may recall to the reader's attention the most important fact that it was not set up by a few schismatics, but by the entire people, with Aaron at their head. The Calf superstition was indubitably in part and

incidentally a relic of what the Israelites had seen in
Egypt in the worship of Apis and Mnevis. Next we
have the golden calves set up by Jeroboam at Dan and
Bethel. Then follows (*Judges* viii. 22, &c.) the worship
of Gideon's Ephod; for the Ephod made by Gideon with
the spoil of the Midianites became after his death an
object of Idolatry. (Lewis, *Orig. Heb.* p. 41.) We have also
Micah's Images and *Teraphim.* The Samaritan temple was
upon Mount Gerizim. " The Jews accuse the Samaritans
of two instances of idolatry committed in this place; the
first, that they worshipped the image of a Dove; the
other that they paid divine adoration to certain Teraphims
or idol gods that were hid under the mountain"—(*Ibid.,*
p. 55). We learn from St. Jerome (who received it by
tradition from the ancient Jews, and indeed it is so stated
in *Numbers,* xxv. 1, 2, &c.—xxiii., 28 and numerous
other passages of the Old Testament,) that the Jews
adored Baal-Phegor (Baal-Pheor), the Priapus of the
Greeks and Romans.—"It was," he says, "principally
worshipped by women—'*colentibus maxime fœminis Baal-
Phegor, ob obscœni magnitudinem quem nos Priapum pos-
sumus appellare.*' "

"The adoration," observes Maimonides, the most
acute and learned of the Cabalistic Doctors, "made to
this idol called Pehor, consisted in *discovering the mons
veneris before it.*" Chemosh (probably the same as Baal-
Pheor) also received the homage of the Jews, as did
Milcom, Molech, Baal-berith (or Cybele), and numerous
others. From all this it will be seen that the Jews fell
into idolatry, and Phallic idolatry too; consequently there
will not appear anything so very startling in the supposition that the Ark of the Covenant contained a Phallus.

We have seen that the *Stone* of Jacob was held in peculiar " veneration," was worshipped and " anointed." We know from the Jewish records that the Ark was sup- posed to contain a *table of stone;* and if it can be demon- strated that that stone was phallic, and yet identical with the sacred name Jehovah or Yehovah, which written in unpointed Hebrew with four letters, is J-E-V-E or J-H-V-H (the H being merely an aspirate and the same as E). This process leaves us the two letters I and V (or in another of its forms U); then if we place the I *in* the U we have the " holy of holies ;" we also have the Linga and Yoni and Argha of the Hindus, the Iswarra or " supreme lord ;" and here we have the whole secret of its mystic and arc-celestial import, confirmed in itself by being identical with the Linyoni of the Ark of the Covenant.

In Gregorie's works [*Notes and Observations upon several Passages in Scripture*—4to, Lond., 1684, vol. i., pp. 120-21] is a passage to the effect that " Noah daily prayed in the Ark before the 'Body of Adam,'" *i.e.* before the Phallus—Adam being the primitive Phallus, great procreator of the human race. " It may possibly seem strange," he says, " that this orison should be daily said before the body of Adam," but "it is a most con- fessed tradition among the eastern men that Adam was commanded by God that his dead body should be kept above ground till a fulness of time should come to commit it פרססאלאוי to the *middle of the earth* by a priest of the Most High God." This means Mount Moriah, the Meru of India.

" This body of Adam was embalmed and transmitted from father to son, till at last it was delivered up by

Lamech into the hands of Noah." Again, "The *middle* of the Ark was the place of prayer, and made holy by the presence of Adam's body." [*Ibid.*, p. 121.] "And so soon as ever the day began to break Noah stood up towards the body of Adam, &c., &c., and prayed."

Here come in the ideas of the Gnostics, and the superstitions concerning "Gallus" and the solemn "cockcrow," the announcement of the morn and the driving back of the darkness, its beaten and discomfited mysterious agents vanishing in the strengthening, magnificent, and yet solemn light, till at last the SUN appears on the rim of the horizon.

To return however to the tables of stone, and to the *Pillar of Jacob.* Our modern rendering of their form is a diagram, or in other words, two headstones placed side by side. Now if we alter the position a little, allowing one to recline horizontally, surmounted by the other perpendicular, we shall obtain a complete Linga and Yoni—the "sacred Name" of the "holy of holies" before mentioned, and the *Pillar* or Mast in the Argha or boat, as represented in the Ark of the Egyptians. The treatment of the Wings of the supporting doves, or sacred birds, on each side of this ark, conveys to us a sufficiently correct idea of where the Hebrews obtained their Cherubim and Seraphim, only substituting a human head and body for the bird's delineation.

Upon consulting the Hebrew dictionary of Gesenius we shall find the word רון (aroun) and ארן (aron) signifying an *ark*, a *chest*. In Genesis l. 26, the word is used as a mummy-chest or coffin for Joseph in Egypt. The ark of the covenant might, in the same way, be called the coffin. For these reasons, it is concluded that the object of veneration in the Ark of the Covenant of the Jews, was a Phallus. It must always be remembered, in all these symbolical and architectural variations, that figurative construction springs from two mathematical forms only. The governing form of all the classic architecture is the horizontal line Thus the Egyptian, the Grecian, the Roman, and all other classic temples are horizontal, oblong, and resemble the *chest*, or "*ark* of the Israelites." On the contrary, the Christian architecture, and that style which the Mahommedans, and the Indians and the Oriental peoples generally, have chosen as typical and indicative of their religious beliefs, takes as its keynote (as we may describe it) the upright, or the perpendicular line. The blending of these, at the intersection or cross-point, forms, of course, the sublime figure indicative of the Christian religion, or the religion of the Cross.

CHAPTER VIII.

IT is observed by Dionysius, the geographer, that Bacchus was worshipped with peculiar zeal and devotion by the ancient inhabitants of some of the smaller British islands. What islands are meant is uncertain; but probably the Hebrides or Orcades. Here the women, crowned with ivy, celebrated his clamorous nocturnal rites upon the shores of the northern ocean, in the same manner as the Thracians did upon the banks of the Absinthus, or the Indians by the Ganges. In Stukeley's *Itinerary* is the ground-plan of an ancient Celtic, or Scandinavian temple, found in Zealand, consisting of a circle of rude stones within a square : and it is probable that many others of these circles were inclosed in square areas. Stonehenge is the most important monument of this kind now extant; and from a passage of Hecatæus, preserved by Diodorus Siculus, it seems to have been not wholly unknown to that ancient historian; who might have collected some vague accounts of the British Islands from the Phœnician and Carthaginian merchants, who traded there for tin. "The Hyperboreans," said he, "inhabit an island beyond Gaul, in which Apollo is worshipped in a circular temple considerable for its size and richness." This island can be no other than Britain.

The large obelisks of stone found in many parts of the

north, such as those at Rudstone and near Boroughbridge
in Yorkshire, belonged to the same religion. Obelisks,
as Pliny observes, were sacred to the Sun; whose rays
they signified both by their form and name. (Lib. xxxvi.,
l. 14.) They were, therefore, the emblems of light, the
primary and essential emanations of the deity; whence
radiating the head, or surrounding it with a diadem of
small obelisks, was a mode of consecration or deification
which flattery often employed in the portraits both of the
Macedemonian kings and of the Roman emperors. The
mystagogues and poets expressed the same meaning by
the epithet ΛΥΚΕΙΟΣ or ΛΥΚΑΙΟΣ; which is occasionally
applied to almost every personification of the deity,
and more especially to Apollo; who is likewise called
ΛΥΚΗΓΕΝΕΤΗΣ, or as contracted, ΛΥΚΗΤΕΝΗΣ; which
mythologists have explained by an absurd fable of his
having been born in Lycia; whereas it signifies the
Author or Generator of Light; being derived from ΛΥΚΗ,
otherwise ΛΥΚΟΣ, of which the Latin word *lux* is a con-
traction. (*Lukeios. Lukaios.—Luké, Lukos.—Il.,* Δ. 101,
Schol. Didym. et Ven. Heraclid. Pant., p. 417, *ed. Gale.*)

In symbolical writing, the same meaning was signified
by the appropriate emblems in various countries; whence
the ΖΕΥΣ ΜΕΙΛΙΧΙΟΣ at Sicyon, and the Apollo Carina
at Megara in Attica, were represented by *stones* of the
above-mentioned form (*Pausan. in Cor.,* c. 9, s. 6); as
was also the Apollo Agyieus in various places; and both
Apollo and Diana by simple columns pointed at the top
(Obelisci or Phalli); or, as the symbol began to be
humanised, with the addition of a head, hands, and feet.
On a Lapland drum, an instrument which was employed
for the purposes of magic and divination, amongst the

consulting mediums of the Lapps and Finns, the goddess appealed to—Isa, or Disa—is represented by a pyramid surmounted with the significant emblem so frequently observed in the hands of the Egyptian deities (*Ol. Rudbeck Atlant.*, p. ii., c. v., p. 277, and c. xi., 261); and the pyramid has likewise been observed among the religious symbols of the savages of North America. (*Lafitau, Mœurs des Sauvages,* t. i., pp. 146 and 8.) The most sacred idol, too, of the Hindoos in the great temple of Juggernaut, in the province of Orissa, is a pyramidal stone (Hamilton's *Travels in India*); and the altar in the temple of Mexico, upon which human victims were sacrificed to the deity of the Sun, was a pointed pyramid, on one side of which the unhappy captive was extended on his back, in order to have his heart taken out by the priest. (Acosta's *History of the Indies,* p. 382.)

The spires and pinnacles with which our old churches are decorated—indeed, all uprights, including all the architectural families, and the varieties of tors, towers, and steeples, the especial mark and glory of Christian building—come from these ancient symbols. They are everywhere indicative of the Phallus, or index-finger denoting the " Fire,"—the aspiring fire, against the inclination of gravity, which was the first vitalised idea, or Idol, worshipped magically and philosophically—the enlivening, godlike Power. The innumerable weathercocks, with which the pointed steeples are surmounted, though now only employed to show the direction of the wind, were originally emblems of the Sun; for the cock is the natural emblem—the magical " look-out," to descry the dawn. The cock, with his "lofty and shrill-sounding cry," in the profundity of the universal stillness, is the natural herald of the day, and therefore sacred to the fountain of light. (*Pausan.*, lib. v., p. 444.) In the symbolical writing of the Chinese, the sun is still represented by a cock in a circle ; and a modern Parsee would suffer death rather than be guilty of the crime of killing one. (*Hyde de Relig. vet. Persarum.*) It appears on many ancient coins, with some symbol of the passive productive power on the reverse (*See coins of Himera, Samothrace, Suessa, &c.*). In some instances it is united with Priapic and other emblems and devices, signifying different attributes combined. (*Ib. and Selinus.*) The Egyptians, among whom of ancient nations the Obelisk and the Pyramid* were the most frequently employed as significant objects, held that there were two opposite powers in the world perpetually acting and reacting against each other; the one generating as the other destroyed ; and the other destroying as fast as the other generated. The former of these powers the Egyptians called Osiris, and the latter, Typhon. By the contention of these two the world was produced, including all the operations of the mind, which was also called "matter," thus agreeing with the realistic contentions of the arch-physicist, Spinoza. By the mutual assistance and inter-action of these two contending Supreme Powers, that mixture of good and evil, of procreation and dissolution, which was to constitute the harmony (necessarily the *balance*) of

---

* The Obelisk always means the male instrument, while the Pyramid signifies the female corresponding tumefactive, or rising power—power not submissive, but answerably suggestive ; synchronised in the anatomical *clitoris*, (root, in the Greek, probably, from *clyte*, "sunflower," as turning to the sun, that eccentric, minute object, meaning everything in the Rosicrucian mystic anatomy.

the world, was supposed to be produced. (*Eurip. apud Plutarch. de Is. et Osir.*) The notion of such a necessary mixture, or reciprocal operation, was, according to Plutarch, of immemorial antiquity, derived from the earliest theologists and legislators, not only in traditions and reports, but also in mysteries and sacred rites, both Greek and Barbarian. (*De Is. et Osir.*, p. 369; *Hippocrat.* Διαιτ., i., 6.) "Fire" was held to be the Efficient Principle of both Powers; that is, the "Light" of Fire was mystically taken as the living power of the Good or Beneficent Impulse; as the "Fire" of Light—the radical base of the same two things, Good, or Light, and Evil, or Fire, was "Fire," motion, heat, or impulse; the whole being simply an abstraction, unintelligible to the mere human reason (which, in reality, as towards God's meanings and purposes, is *nothing*); the two contrarieties or opposites being, in fact, the same thing, out of the mind, and independent not only of phenomena, but, farther, of the possibility of phenomena. This is the true doctrine—abstract, and hopelessly mystical as it is—of the Rosicrucians, which has been universally misunderstood by the learned world, and shrunk from by Christian theologians. According to some of the later Egyptians, the ethereal fire was supposed to be concentrated in the sun. But Plutarch controverts this opinion, and asserts that Typhon, the evil or destroying power, was a terrestrial or material fire, essentially different from the æthereal. Plutarch means that the æthereal or celestial Fire is "Light," which is the flower, the glory, or *acmé* of Heat, stimulated into visibility, lucidity, into proof of itself, into Fire. Plutarch, as well as other Greek writers, admits Typhon to have been the brother of Osiris, the Cain to the Abel, Esau to the Jacob, "Law" to the "Prophets," *Omega* to *Alpha* of the Judaic or Israelitish system. The Greeks regarded this "Dark Genius" as a being as sacred in his own way as the "Genius of the Light," equally sprung from κρονος and ρεα, or Time and Matter. In this, however, as in other instances, he followed his own prepossessions, and was partly led by the new system of the Egyptian Platonics (Gnosticism, in fact), according to which there was an Original Evil Principle in nature, co-eternal with the Good, and acting in perpetual opposition to it. This opinion owes its origin to a false notion, which we are apt to form of good and evil, by considering them as self-existing inherent properties, instead of relative modifications dependent upon circumstances and causes. We owe the very capacity for thinking about good and evil at all, or of knowing any difference in them, to the fact that *in the abstract*, in nature, there is really no difference between good and evil.

The arrow or dart (βελος, or οβελος), was the appropriate emblem of the power that was exercised by the "Fire," Sun, Apollo or Phœbus. Every Obelisk was a typical representative in stone of a ray or beam of the far-darting, operative, vivifying fire. If the obelisks are attentively regarded, apart from the ornamental cradles in which they are deposited, it will be seen that they have no squared, solidly-imposed bases; but that the angles are rounded, or orbicular, with the intention that the whole ponderous weight should rest on a centre thread line, with the liberty to poise, or oscillate, or swing freely. This was the intention in the mind of the original fabricators and setters-up of these monster magic splints of stone; they were raised to nod or bow intelligently, recognising and replying magically, as oracles, to questions on the part of superstitious consultants—like the modern "tipping tables" of the Spiritualists. These ideas of the value set upon them, and of the respect and supernatural awe with which they were regarded, seem natural enough when we remember the strange and hitherto unintelligible name by which they were known among the early people in Wales and Cornwall—that of "Bowing-Stones"—and when we can see with our own eyes how such rolling and swinging on their own axes when first set moving in oscillation, was possible to these stupendous, giddy monsters. The obelisks would thus prove of the same original purpose as the "Logan," or Rocking-Stones. These were overpowering masses so beautifully poised as to be capable of being set in motion by the finger of a child—consultant Idols of Stone, into which the "Logh," or Spirit of God, was supposed to descend, when invoked, in the assembly of the people seeking answers from the Deity, and prostrated before the majestically sublime, supposed enchanted object.

The signs of the zodiac were taken from the mystic symbols; and not, as some learned authors have supposed, the mystic symbols from the signs of the zodiac. By attracting or heaving the waters of the ocean, the Moon (Diana) naturally appeared to be the sovereign of humidity; and by seeming to operate so powerfully upon the constitutions of women, she equally appeared to be the patroness and regulatress of nutrition and passive generation. "Calor solis ære facit, lunaris humectat." (*Macrob., Sat.* vii., c. x.) The ancient Egyptians, or at least some of them, appear to have known that water and air are but of one substance. (*Plutarch de Is. et Osir.*)

There is vast ignorance, after all, in the ideas of contemporary commentators upon the architectural monuments of the Egyptians, and as we fully believe, a total, sublimely unconscious misreading, and failure at comprehension, of the real meanings of the hieroglyphics—*an imagined translation of which is so ostentatiously paraded by those supposedly able professors.*

Some of these verbose critics—overwhelming us with a prodigious and apparently inexhaustible deluge of talk—are apt to confound personages for the purpose of contracting dates. Warburton has humorously introduced one of these clever chronologers, proving that William the Conqueror and William the Third were one and the same person. (*Div. Leg.*) History, in reality, has suffered most from the historians.

The earliest capital, in that which is called the classic architecture, seems to have been the bell, or seed-vessel, simply copied, without any alteration, except a little expansion, at bottom, to give it stability. The Egyptian architecture appears to have been original and indigenous, and in this art only the Greeks seem to have borrowed from them, the different orders being only different modifications of the symbolical columns which the Egyptians formed in imitation of the *nelumbo,* the lotus or water-lily. Columns and capitals of the same kind are still existing, in great numbers, among the ruins of Thebes in Egypt; and more particularly among those on the island of Philæ on the borders of Æthiopia, which was anciently held so sacred that none but priests were permitted to go upon it. The Ionic capital has no bell, but volutes formed in imitation of sea-shells, which have the same symbolical meaning. To these architectural ad-

juncts is frequently added the ornament which architects
call the honeysuckle. The Greeks decorated the capitals
of their columns with the foliage of various plants, sometimes of the *acanthus*, and sometimes of the aquatic kind.
(*See Denon.*, pl. lix., 1, 2, and 3, and lx., 1, 2, 3, &c.,
where the originals from which the Greeks took their
Corinthian capitals plainly appear.) It might have been
more properly called the "Egyptian" order, so far at
least as relates to the form and decoration of the capitals.
Peculiar decorative mouldings, of exceeding grace and
beauty, are introduced in the Ionic order, among which
figure largely the honeysuckle and lotus. Another enrichment is also employed, in graceful combination, in the
capitals and mouldings. This is architectural detail, in the
mouldings, full of suggested purpose, and called the "egg
and anchor," or "egg and tongue," (adder's-tongue),
and "spear-head" mouldings. On the Isiac table, the
figures of Isis are represented holding the stem of the
lotus, surmounted by the seed-vessel in one hand and the
circle and cross (the *crux ansata*) in the other. All the
Greek architecture bears the tokens of the Egyptian,
rendered elegant.

We may reasonably infer that the greatest number of the
superb edifices now remaining in Egypt, were executed,
or at least begun, before the Homeric, or even Trojan
times; many of them being such as could not have been
finished but in a long course of years, even supposing the
wealth and resources of the ancient kings of Egypt to
have equalled those of the greatest of the Roman emperors.
The columns being thus sacred symbols, the temples
themselves, of which they always formed the principal
part, were emblems of the deity, signifying generally the

passive productive power. Thus the classic styles of
architecture, the Greek and the Roman, and particularly
that of the lateral (*arca*, "ark-like," "archaic," meaning
old), or tabernacle, of which the horizontal line of the
Cross was the sacred symbol, meaning mystically the
"To-Be," or the "Jussit," of the Infinite Contriver of
All—or to speak masonically, the "Great Architect of
the Universe," the King (of Kings), or the "Great
Master :"—the classic temples, we repeat, were always
figured forth, or detailed, in the lateral or universal horizontal or fluent base-line, unceiled ("sealed"), open to
the heavens, from which the divinity was supposed to
descend to his shrine. All this was reproduced in certain
ways in the Christian system, and particularly in the
Gnostic readings of christianity.

The most obvious and consequently the most ancient
symbol of the productive power of the "Waters" (the
"Great Deep," the "Second Person in the Universe,"
the "Second Person of the Christian Trinity"), in the
mystic sense, the Chr-ist (**X**) or the Virgin Mary,
(*Maria, Mar, Mare*), either divinity, indifferently, from
the *feminine angle* as the point of view—the most ancient
of the symbols of the second great power of the Rosicrucians, we repeat, was a fish. The ancients, particularly
the Phœnicians, *barbarised* this idea, parodying it, although
seriously and intentionally, into their Dagon, or God of
the Great Deep, or the Waters.*

* From this acceptation of the myth we obtain the " Waters divided
from the Waters" of the Mosaic theosophical cosmogony—the
" Abyss," the matter out of which all things were made, and "without
which nothing was made," of the philosophers—the Deluge, or the
extinction of all guilty humanity in the divine judgment—the Ark, or

We find the universal symbol, the Fish (*Icthius, Ix-theus*), Ix-ion, (the Rock), the Fish, as the Gnostic symbol of the Saviour in many ways, upon many of the earliest coins. It is a principal figure upon the Gnostic gems or talismans. The goddess of the Phœnicians was repre-sented by the head and body of a woman, terminating below in a fish. (*Lucian de Syr. Dea*, s. 14.) But on the Phœnician as well as Greek coins, now extant, the personage is of the other sex. And in plate L. of vol. i. of the Select Specimens is engraved a beautiful figure of the mystic Cupid or first-begotten Love, terminating in an aquatic plant which, affording more elegance and variety of form, was employed to signify the same mean-ing—that is, the "Spirit upon the Waters." From this connexion of ideas between the Fish and the Saviour, comes the mystic symbol meaning the female *vulva* or fish's mouth—the mitre, cleft and peculiarly shaped, of the archbishops and bishops, especially those examples of the very earliest Christian mitres, or the cloven, sym-bolical, sacred head-coverings. The fur *Pileus*, Pileon,

---

the preservation of the example of humanity through Noah—the Raven of Doom, the " black flying spirit of condemnation :"—the Dove with wings but without feet, " no rest for the sole of her foot" (the original of the younger sons' martlet in heraldry), the white, re-soaring, angel-winged spirit of reconciliation, and of the second dispensation, and of forgive-ness and new life, accorded through the woman as the means of the Holy-Sex. This the female is, and thus blessed by God-Almighty and committed to the guardianship of Man—for whom (mystically) he stands responsible to God in his " First-Death," although *not* in his " Second"—for in the spiritual acceptance of the idea of Death, there are " Two Deaths." All life dies the First Death. It is to be hoped that very few have died or will die the " Second Death"—regarding which, we have mystical hints in the unexplored pro-fundities of Scripture.

or black or dark-coloured rough coronal, worn by corporate officers, as well as the military, Tartar or Oriental
light-horse (skirmishing horse), *fur* head-covers, with the
dangling "fly" or tail (there ought properly to be *two*), are
Ismaelitish, irregular, bastard (grandly-bastard, for what
they mean) proofs of this special magical swarthy service,
or devotion to the Venus of the people (Venus Pandemos), or the original grand "Hussey"—to speak of her
by the popular old English term—or general strumpet.
In reality, this mystic original is taken for the "Mother
of the Nations"—the Female Dark-Doer—the *Hetaira*,
Hagar—producer of the left-handed side of the population, and a true benefactress of the race human in the
freedom of her favours. Her aggressive, warlike priests—
a sort of *corybanti*, with their Moresco bells or jingles, the
Oriental or Mahometan reproduction of the paraphernalia
of the classic "clash and clamour"—by cymbals, voice,
and bells—a sort of "Bacchic rout," only, like the
Cossacks, careering and shouting their "*huzzas*" (from
which comes the name Hussar, both from Uza, Venus,
or Hussey),—are the regiments of Light Cavalry, Pandours, or Hussars, employed as marauders, a sort of
military wasps or hornets. In the word Pandours
(Hungarian Light Cavalry of this sprightly, fiercely mischievous kind), notice the *Pan* as indicative of the
"Touch-and-Go" — "everywhere" — of their style
of active carrying-on of this military game of sinister,
although, from their system and their horseman-
ship and their trappings, graceful and picturesque
annoyance. [See the "ROSICRUCIANS," Second Edition, pp. 255—258, for full proofs of the mysteriously eccentric origin of the Light Irregular Cavalry

of all western armies, as exemplified in their equipments.]

Virginity was a something especially looked upon as inalienable, and as a particular property of the Gods. It was a supernatural gift—out of the liabilities, and independent of the world. No mortal dared touch it. Savage barbarism only could lay hand on it. Thus, even the Bride was, in certain regards, *only a victim.* Hence her investment in *white* was as much a penitential denotement as an indication of purity. The victims, among the Romans, were arrayed in white. She was to be *snatched,* as it were, from her relatives for the purpose of marriage; hence the pretended "running away" with the Bride, with the masquerading exhibition of the "violent hand," on the part of the Bridegroom, to seize her, amongst some early peoples. For these reasons, the Roman nation entertained some very awful, superstitious ideas, in their profound respect for the magic defensiveness and sacred putting aside implied in the very name of virgin.*

* Hence the duties of the Best-Man in the celebration of a marriage; very fortunately alleviated in modern times, otherwise we should find very few (even devoted friends) disposed to accept such serious and uncomfortable responsibilities. The "Best-Man" was the intended Husband's Champion. He was bound in the old rigorous day, by oath, to deliver the "Betrothed One," or the Bride, spotless and safe, into the hands of the Bridegroom, his "liege-principal" on the occasion. It was the obligation of this Best-Man to become the armed sentinel, and to take post before the Bedchamber-Door, then become sacred and solemn, where what was to be done was to be done in the presence of the Gods (*solvere zonam, &c.*). The Best-Man, fully armed and equipped—in ancient times it was in armour, with visor down (for the champion was anonymous),—kept guard before the door; and since to him was committed possession of the key (in copy of the "symbol" key), he had, sword in hand, to maintain the door or doors against all comers; vitally against those who might attempt

The chastity of the Vestal Virgins—who had charge of the "Holy Fire"—equally as the virginity of the Nuns of Saint Bridget among the earlier devotees of the Christian faith, who, with a like observance, maintained "sentry" —Amazon-Priests, as they might be called, in this manner —over the undying "Light" in the cloisters and sanctuaries of the Christ:—this state of absolute virginity was an all-powerful object. No matter what the enormity of her guilt otherwise, the woman—if a virgin—could not be subjected to the last penalty of death by violent hand. Here we see the reason of the "putting away"— or the silent, awful, living burial of the Vestal Virgin, even in the doubt—no one having witnessed the act—of

rescue. The sentry's duty was to keep this watch until daydawn, when his particular service was supposed to be superseded or accomplished. It was defensive duty of this kind which was imagined to be the origin of "pledging," for safety at convivial meetings. The purpose and use has in modern days, and in the exercise of modern formalities, passed altogether out of recognition or of knowledge. This singular watch of the Bridegroom's "Best-Man" was held in full solemnity until the sentinel was relieved at "cock-crow," when his obligations were terminated. Any attempts at disturbance (for the women, amongst the ancients, used to make a show of rushing to the assistance of the Bride) or at interruption—even on the part of the most desperate rival of the newly-married man, who, at all hazards, wanted to break in—for such things have occurred—were to be resolutely withstood whilst the sentry remained the custodian of the "key," and he was compelled to hold his post, and, if necessary, to slay his assailant, even although he should be his own brother. And also, in this extremity, he would be held harmless, his full justification (by law both Divine and human) being the fact that the Bridal-Chamber was a holy place, as it was mystically "sealed and sacred," both as regards men and spirits ; and that he was bound, even at the risk of his life, to keep guard over it, in the due discharge of this high chivalric function. We here recall some mystical doings, even in the ceremonies of the Freemasons, in the proper observances of their sublime forms in the sealed lodge.

the infraction of her vows ;—and the evidence being
presumptive only of her guilt. Hence the fine precautions
of the Roman equity. As a singular difference, in the
ideas of the strange sacredness, and also the peculiar
religious perfection even of the idea of the *want* of
virginity amongst different peoples, in the contrariety of
their superstition, may be cited the impressions of the
Hindoos. In the minds of this people, no woman is a fit
candidate for Heaven unless she has fulfilled what to them is
the very purpose of her being, and sacrificed her virginity;
made over, as it were, her due to God—no female enter-
ing Heaven who seeks to pass bodily unproven. Such a
notion prevailed, also, among the Israelites :—witness the
lament for Tammaz or Thammaz, the Hebrew "Phœbus,"
and the period of sacrificial "mourning amidst the mountains," spent by the daughter of Jephtha—a sort of
Iphigenia—"*bewailing her virginity;*" and this actually
"before the Lord." This is one of the most tragical and
touching stories in the Old Testament narrative, to the
meanings of which very little attention is ordinarily paid.
The Mahometans imagine that woman has no soul, and
therefore no place in a future world, unless qualified and
fitted therefor by being taken out of the ordinary cate-
gory of women by extra-natural means, and by special
magic merits. The *Houris*—the female, exquisitely
physically endowed populace of the Mussulman Paradise
—the Spirit Flowers of which are only for plucking and
renewing use, are merely impersonated means of aggressive
male delight.

A writer* who makes very nice distinctions in these

* Pierre Dufour, *L'Antiquité la plus reculée jusqu'à nos jours*,
vol. iii., chap. i., Bruxelles, 1861.

important respects, has the following :—" Voilà pourquoi, pendant les persécutions, il y eut tant de vierges chré-tiennes* outragées par leurs bourreaux, qui ne faisaient qu'appliquer l'antique loi romaine, en vertu de laquelle une vierge ne pouvait pas être mise à mort." " Les Juges Païens prenaient un odieux plaisir à les frapper dans ce qu'elles avaient de plus cher. Mais leur virginité était un sacrifice qu'elles offraient chastement à Dieu en échange de la couronne du martyre. ' Une vierge,' disait Saint-Ambroise, ' peutêtre prostituée et non souillée.' ' Les vierges,' dit Saint-Cyprien, ' sont comme les fleurs du Jardin de Ciel.' " And when forced, the author might have added, they become still more glorious flowers, or lights, of Paradise.

The reason for all this lies very deep, and is very refined and true. It will be readily seen on reflection that, owing to these ideas of the inherent sacredness of virginity (although, without the infraction of it, the human world could, of course, not be), the execu-tioners of the heathen nations were debarred from their incontestable right of public execution in the case of delinquent females, whether virgin or otherwise, were it not that in their superstitious reverence, they dared not " outrage" their gods by touching their property, as it were. In the fine devotional sensibility prevailing amongst

---

* " *Outragées par leurs bourreaux.*"

" *Boult.* How's this ? We must take another course with you. . . . Come your ways.

Marina. Whither would you have me ?

Boult. I must have your virtue taken off, *or the common hangman shall execute it.* Come your ways. We'll have no more gentlemen driven away. Come your ways, I say."—*Pericles, Prince of Tyre,* Act IV., Scene 6.

the people, therefore, by the Roman law the *carnificæ*, or executioners, were compelled, before they destroyed them (so curiously to express the idea), to eliminate the "god" out of the victim before they inflicted the last penalty; and they consequently were obliged, as a part of their odious office, indeed as their duty, to deflower the females; and in plucking the last beautiful, dear "Rose" of their maidenhood out of them, to make them *things*, fit to be thrown away.*

This is the reason why, according to the old unwritten law of England, ancient as the foundations of the Constitution itself, women, in the hands of the public executioners, were always burned or strangled at the stake, and thus dismissed as it were honourably, and not hanged, like men or dogs. It was a tribute to the supposed God in *woman* as the more glorious and magic object; and it was an acknowledgment of the supposed sacredness of the strangely mysterious characteristics in the arrangements of the mystic anatomy, wherein she is specially constituted, with nevertheless singular drawbacks, disabilities, and peculiarities. Man is philosophically held to be a phenomenon, just as woman is regarded as a phenomenon, only, in the latter case, to an infinitely farther extent. From some of these reasons arises the inherent sacredness of the human "Act" all the world over, and highest and most profoundly so in the religions of the most civilised peoples.

---

* "Le viol des vierges chrétiennes n'était donc dans l'origine qu'un préliminaire de la peine capitale, conformément à l'usage de la pénalité romaine. 'Vitiatæ prius a carnifice, dein strangulatæ.'" (Suetonius *dans la vie de Tibère*).—Pierre Dufour, *L'Histoire de Prostitution.*

CHAPTER IX.

THE PHALLI, AND THE OPHIOLOGICAL PRIAPIC MONUMENTS,
TYPICAL OF "THE FALL."

THERE were piles of stones, or single stones, distributed in former times all over the north, called by the
Greeks ΛΟΦΟΙ 'ΕΡΜΑΙΟΙ, little hills, or mounds of Mercury;
of whom they were probably the original symbols. They
were placed by the sides, or in the points of intersection,
of roads ; and every traveller that passed (" *Siste, viator,*")
threw a stone upon them in honour of Mercury, the
guardian of all ways, or the general classic conductor.
(*Anthol.,* lib. iv., Epigr. 12; *Phurnut. de Nat. Deor.*)
There can be no doubt that many of the ancient Crosses
observable in such situations were erected upon these
mounds, their pyramidal form affording a commodious
base, and the substitution of a new object being the most
obvious and usual remedy for such kinds of superstition.

The old Pelasgian Mercury of the Athenians consisted
of a human head placed upon an inverted obelisk with a
phallus ; of which several are extant. We find also female
draped figures terminating in the same square form. These
seem to be of the Venus Architis, or Primitive Venus ;
of whom there was a statue of wood at Delos, supposed
to be the work of Dædalus ; and another in a temple upon
Mount Libanus, of which the description of Macrobius
exactly corresponds with the figures now extant. Her
appearance was melancholic, her head covered, and her
face sustained by her left hand, which was concealed
under her garment. (Sat. i., chap. xxi.) Some of these

figures have the mystic title ΑΣΠΑΣΙΑ upon them, signifying perhaps the welcome or gratulation to the returning spring: for they evidently represent nature in winter, still sustained by the inverted obelisk, the emanation of the sun pointed downwards but having all her powers enveloped in gloom and sadness. Some of these figures were probably, like the Paphian Venus, androgynous; whence arose the *Hermaphroditæ*, afterwards represented under more elegant forms; accounted for as usual by poetical fables. Occasionally the attribute seems to be signified by the cap and wings of Mercury.

The symbolical meaning of the olive, the fir, and the apple, the honorary rewards in the Olympic, Isthmian, and Pythian games, all bore reference to the myths, and the mysteries in religion. The parsley, which formed the crown of the Roman victors, was equally a mystic plant; it being represented on coins in the same manner as the fig-leaf, and with the same signification (*Hesych :*), probably on account of a peculiar influence which it is still supposed to have upon the female constitution.

The confusion of personages and of characteristics among the gods and heroes, arising from a confusion of names and terms, was facilitated in its progress by the belief that the universal generative principle, or its subordinate emanations, might act in such a manner that a female of the human species might be impregnated without the co-operation of a male. (*Plutarch. Symposiac*, lib. viii., probl. 1.) And as this notion was extremely useful and convenient in concealing the frailties of women, quieting the jealousies of husbands, protecting the honour of families, and guarding with religious awe the power of bold usurpers, it was naturally cherished and promoted with much favour and industry. Men were supposed to be produced in this supernatural way. Even the double or ambiguous sex was attributed to deified heroes; Cecrops being fabled to have been both man and woman.*

Among the rites and customs of the temple at Hieropolis, that of the priests castrating themselves, and assuming the manners and attire of women (as the women of the temple disguised themselves as men sometimes) is one of the most unaccountable. The same customs prevailed in Phrygia among the priests and priestesses of Cybelè and Attis. They, perhaps, arose from a notion of being made emblematic of the Deity by acquiring an androgynous appearance. It is possible, likewise, that the male devotees might have concluded that a deprivation of virility was the best incentive to that spiritual enthusiasm, to which women were observed to be more liable than men; and to which all sensual indulgence, particularly that of the sexes (although the opportunities therefor, from these circumstances, were most convenient), was held to be peculiarly adverse. The ancient German prophetesses, who exercised such unlimited control over a people who would submit to no human authority, were virgins consecrated to the Deity, like the Roman Vestals. (*See Tacit. de M. G.*)

The similarity of the religious systems of India and of Egypt is so great, that it is impossible to doubt that they arose from the same source. One of the most remarkable parallels in the usages springing from theosophical ideas prevailing in Hindostan, and in the land of the

---

* *Justin*, lib. ii., c. 6; *Suidas.*, *Euseb. et Hieron. in Chronic.*; *Plutarch. de sera numin. vindicta.*; *Eustath. in Dionys.*; *Diodor. Sic.*, l. i., c. 28.

Pharaohs, is the hereditary division into castes, derived from *metempsychosis.* This doctrine formed the rule, and was a fundamental article of faith in both India and Egypt, as also with the ancient Gauls, Britons, and many other nations. The Hindoo castes rank according to the number of transmigrations which the soul is supposed to have undergone, and its consequent proximity to, or distance from, re-absorption into the divine essence, or intellectual abyss, from which it sprang. The sacred Brahmins, whose souls are approaching to a re-union with their source, are far above the wretched pariahs, who are lowest in the alphabet of *castes.* These last are without any rank in the hierarchy; and are therefore supposed to have all the long, humiliating, and painful transmigrations yet before them. As the respective distinctions are, in both, hereditary, the soul being supposed to descend into one class for punishment and ascend into the other for reward, the misery of degradation is without hope even in posterity; the wretched parents having nothing to bequeath to their unfortunate offspring that is not tainted with everlasting infamy and humiliation. Loss of *caste* is therefore the most dreadful punishment that a Hindoo can suffer; as it affects both his body and his soul, extends beyond the grave, and reduces both him and his posterity for ever to a situation below that of a brute.

From the specimens that have appeared in European languages, the poetry of the Hindoos seems to be in the same style as their art; and to consist of gigantic, gloomy, and operose fictions, destitute of all those graces which distinguish the religious and poetical fables of the Greeks.

The incarnations which form the principal subjects of

sculpture in all the temples of India, Tibet, Tartary, and China, are above all others calculated to call forth the ideal perfections of the art, by expanding and exalting the imagination of the artist, and exciting his ambition to surpass the simple imitation of ordinary forms, in order to produce a model of excellence worthy to be the corporeal habitation of the Deity: but this, no nation of the East, nor indeed of the Earth, except the Greeks and those who copied them, ever attempted. Let the precious wrecks and fragments, therefore, of the art and genius of that wonderful people be " collected with care and preserved with reverence," as examples of what man is capable of under peculiar circumstances; which, as they have never occurred but once, may never occur again !

After the supreme Triad, the framers of the vast Oriental system supposed an immense host of inferior spirits to have been produced; part of whom afterwards rebelling under their chiefs Moisasoor and Rhaabon, the material world was prepared for their prison and place of purgation; in which they were to pass through " eighty-nine transmigrations" prior to their restoration. During this time they are exposed to the machinations of their former leaders; who endeavour to make them violate the laws of the Omnipotent, and thus relapse into hopeless perdition, or lose their *caste,* and have all the tedious and painful transmigrations already passed to go through again; to prevent which, their more dutiful brethren, the Emanations that remained faithful to the Omnipotent, were allowed to comfort, cherish, and assist them in their passage: and that all might have equal opportunities of redeeming themselves, the Divine Personages of the " Great Triad" (the same, in efficacy and purpose, as the Christian "Trinity,") had at different times become incarnate in different forms (the Christian system of " Mercy," or of " Mediation" or " Redemption"), and in different countries, to the inhabitants of which they had given different laws and institutions suitable to their respective climates, natures, and circumstances. It would follow from this, that each religion may be good, and may be efficacious in the furtherance of the Divine ultimate intentions, of which, of course, Man must be entirely ignorant; and in regard of which, he may make complete mistakes, from the insufficiency of that which he assumes to be *reason;* while of absolute truth man knows nothing; or why can he not foresee the future just as he recalls the past?

The head of Proserpine appears, in numberless instances, surrounded by dolphins. And upon the very ancient medals of Sidè in Pamphylia, the pomegranate, the fruit peculiarly consecrated to her, is borne upon the back of one. (*Mus. Hunter.*, tab. xlix., fig. 3, &c.) By prevailing upon her to eat of pomegranate, Pluto is said to have procured her stay during half the year in the infernal regions; and a part of the Greek ceremony of marriage still consists, in many places, in the bride's treading upon a pomegranate. The flower of it is also occasionally employed as an ornament upon the diadems of both Hercules and Bacchus, and likewise forms the device of the Rhodian medals; on some of which we have seen distinctly represented an ear of barley springing from one side of it, and the bulb of the lotus, or nelumbo, from the other. It therefore holds the place of the male, or active generative attribute; and accordingly we find it on a bronze fragment published by Caylus, as the result of the union of the bull and lion, exactly as the more distinct symbol of the phallus is in a similar fragment above cited. (*Recueil d'Antiquités,* &c., vol. vii., pl. lxiii., figs. 1, 2, and 3.) The pomegranate, therefore, in the hand of Proserpine or Juno, signifies the same as the circle and cross, before explained, in the hand of Isis; which is the reason why Pausanias declines giving any explanation of it, lest it should lead him to divulge any of the mystic secrets of his religion. (*Corinth.,* c. xvii., s. 4.) The cone of the pine, with which the thyrsus of Bacchus is always surmounted, and which is employed in various compositions, is probably a symbol of similar import.

Those caps resembling the *Petasus* of Mercury explain its purpose, and its significance, guarded, however, effectually in the injunctions of the mythological *Harpocrates* (the everlasting "protector of the mysteries"—the Great Sentinel, or Tiler of the Freemasons); who holds the guards of the "Triple Lodge" of the Heavens above, the "Earth" in the midst, "between the Waters and the Waters," and the "Under Regions." *

These caps, the *Petasi,* Phrygian Caps of the mystic

---

* The mystic authority of this inexorable officer, or Grand Guard, stretching, in imagination, over the "Three Worlds," and emblemed in his trenchant, bared glaive, which, in reality, is typical of the Sword of Saint Michael. We see this weapon figured in the arms of the Corporation of the City of London, in the upper chief quarter, or *canton* (as the Heralds call it), as the Sword of Saint Paul. In popular acceptation, this is the dagger wherewith Sir William Walworth despatched the rebel, Wat Tyler; Wat Tyler however was only struck down by the mace of the Lord Mayor, then, of course, in full panoply of his knight's plate-mail; and was despatched by the dagger, or *misericorde,* of one of the King's own Knights in attendance; whose name is not recorded, and who certainly never popularly obtained the honour of killing Richard the Second's most formidable enemy.

fiery purification, " the form of which is derived from the egg," says Payne Knight,* " and which are worn by the Dioscuri" (*Di-oscuri,* the secret, dark, or unknown gods), " as before observed, surmounted with asterisks, signify the hemispheres of the earth. (*Sext. Empiric.,* xi., 37; see also *Achill. Tat. Isagog.,* p. 127 b. and 130 c.) And it is possible that the asterisks may, in this case, mean the morning and evening stars."

The cap is the Isiac, or Memphian, thrice-sacred head-cover, and is the origin of the united " king-priestly" mitre, the diadem of the Persian monarchs, as also of the mythic hood of the Doges of Venice, or the " coronet-encircled" crown, with the bulged salient cap—cloven, in the instance of the Emperors of the East and the West in Europe, those of Russia and of Germany.

Both " destruction" and " creation" were, according to the religious philosophy of the ancients, merely " disso-lution" and " renovation;" to which all sublunary bodies, even that of the Earth itself, were supposed to be periodi-cally liable. " Fire" and " water" were held to be the great efficient principles of both; and as the spirit or vital principle of thought and mental perception was alone supposed to be immortal and unchanged, the complete dissolution of the body, which it animated, was conceived to be the only means of its complete emancipation. Herein

---

* Payne Knight evidently did not know that this mythic cap, or cover for the head—called, in modern times, the " Cap of Liberty"—and which is always *red,* means the Sacrificial Rite of Circumcision. " Whence this Cap," he observes, " became a distinction of rank, as it was among the Scythians (πιλοφορικοι, ' *Scythians of rank,*' Lucian. *Scyth.*), or ' a symbol of freedom and emancipation,' as it was among the Greeks and Romans, is not easily ascertained. (See *Tib. Hemsterhuis., Not. in Lucian. Dialog. Deor.,* xxi.)"

the doctrines of the Budd*h*ists (or B*h*uddists, which latter is the more proper accentuation,) precisely agree with the ideas of the Greeks and Romans. The Egyptian monarchs erected for the final deposition of their own bodies those vast pyramidal monuments (the symbols of that " Fire" of which they were commemorative), whose excessive strength and solidity were well calculated to secure them as long as the earth itself lasted.

The corporeal residence of this divine particle or emanation, the soul, as well as of the grosser principle of vital heat and animal motion, was supposed to be the blood. Hence the ever-reappearing ideas of the *sacred character of the blood*, prevailing in all the theologies which have learning for their base; and notably amongst the Orientals (the Hebrews, particularly), the Greeks, the Romans, and even the Christians, in the delicacy of their profounder philosophical learning, as indicated in their ideas of the " mystic processes" of the Crucifixion, the Holy Eucharist, and the deep meanings of the order of the " Round Table," and concentrating around the ideas of the " Red Cross," and the " Roses."

Purification by fire is still in use among the Hindoos, as it was among the earliest Romans, and also among the native Irish; men, women, and children, and even cattle, in Ireland, leaping over, or passing through the sacred fires annually kindled in honour of Baal; an ancient title of the Sun, or rather of the " Celestial Fire"—the last thing to be penetrated to (in magic) of all created things.

To this idea of sacrifice, and to the expiatory sacrifice in blood, we owe the compositions, so frequent in the sculptures of the third and fourth centuries, of Mithras, the Persian Mediator, or his female personification, a winged Victory, sacrificing a bull. It seems probable that the sanctity anciently attributed to red or purple arose from its similitude to blood, for it had been customary, in early times, to paint not only the faces of the statues of the deities with vermilion (properly *carmine*), but also the bodies of the Roman Consuls and Dictators, during the sacred ceremony of the Triumph; from which ancient custom the imperial purple of later ages is derived.

. From these ideas of the magic and the sacredness of colours, particularly in the augurial and heraldic sense, it is apparent that the ancient augurs were heralds. The modern heralds are, or ought to be, rightfully, augurs in certain illustrative respects, in regard to the due marshalling of arms in the mystic or *meaning* sense. Red is the royal colour. Purple is the imperial colour, as meaning the union of royalties, or the Greater Kingship, or the title of "King of Kings." The richest blood has a purplish tinge, as is well known. From this reason, comes the very little understood word "blue-blood" (*sang-azur*), as implying the true, pure aristocracy. Therefore, in the mystic and mythological sacred inflection, whilst Jupiter becomes the King of the Gods and claims red, or instant, or simple blood-colour, as his distinguishing colour, the anarch, or earliest of the Gods, or father of Jupiter, or as he may be designated, in this connection, the Emperor of the Gods—Saturn, has assigned for arch-kingly, or *imperial* colour, the exquisitely-heightened blood-colour, in deepest dignity, or purple. The real Tyrian purple, as it is called, was not absolutely red, as by most mistaken historians it is assumed to have been, but a *carmine*, of inexpressible brilliancy and beauty. The tinge of this truly majestic colour, and its mysterious means of production, are, with the true composition of the celebrated Greek Fire of the ancient times, and the mode of hammering glass as a metal, and using this brittle solidity as a means of constructing fabrics, registered among the lost arts. And these and similar are rejected in the modern scientific self-satisfaction, and laughed at as being, in the contemporaneous estimate, impossible: as impossible as the ever-burning lamps, or other marvels dreamed about, written about, or talked about.

Bells and jingles are always part of the paraphernalia among the Follies, Fees, or Fays; Mimes or Tom-Fools flocking out to mischief and merriment in the Festivals, Carnivals, and Pantomimes sacred or secular. These and such have figured, in all the historical ages, in all countries, from the classic times until the present. They are equally to the front in our own day, as every one knows. But these fanciful ideas, involving the careering of both classes of priests and priestesses—real Bacchantes and Bacchanals—in grand parade, and with all the customary celebration of Priapic usages, are much better understood, and infinitely more picturesquely and artistically celebrated and represented, with greatly more art, address, and taste, in Paris and Vienna, than in London.

Many Priapic figures of the old times (still extant) have bells attached to them (*Bronzi d'Ercolano*, t. vi., tav. xcviii.), as the symbolical statues and temples of the Hindoos have; and to wear them was a part of the worship of Bacchus among the Greeks (*Megasthen. apud Strab.*, lib. xv., p. 712), whence we sometimes find them of extremely small size, evidently meant to be worn as amulets, with the *phalli, lunulæ,* &c. The chief priests of the Egyp-

H

tians, and also the high priest of the Jews, hung these bells, as sacred emblems, to their sacerdotal garments; and the Brahmins still continue to ring a small bell at the intervals of their prayers, ablutions, and other acts of mystic devotion; which custom is still preserved in the Catholic Church at the elevation of the host. (*Plutarch. Symposiac.*, lib. iv., qu. 5; *Exod.*, c. xxviii.) The Lacedemonians beat upon a brass vessel or pan—a kettle-drum; which idea was, perhaps, the origin of the "kettle-drums" solely pertaining to the Household Cavalry of the Sovereign of England, and covered with the banners, or trophies, of the royal arms. The Lacedemonians, as a mystic observance, or ceremony in honour of their gods, beat upon these metallic discs, or drums, on the death of their kings. We still retain the custom of tolling a bell on such occasions. The Chinese raise a clash amidst their metals, at the time of an eclipse, in order, as they say, to scare away the "Great Dragon," which has laid a plot to carry away the light—his great enemy, the "Dragon Slayer," Phœbus, the Sun.

The reason of these parallel ceremonies, among all the peoples, and the singular similarity of their superstitions, locally and generally, as if they, with one consent, were addressed to the same object, with only slightly varying manners; and the use made, apparently, of the self-same machinery to work towards these ends, remain as generally unknown as ever, in spite of innumerable guesses. The *raison d'être* of ancient ceremonies which still survive, and their obstinate adherence and tenacity in the usage, even in the affections of the people,—the inherent life of superstitions, surprises us, whilst they, in truth, bewilder.

"It is said," says the Golden Legend by Wynkyn

de Worde, "the evil spirytes that ben in the regyon of th' ayre doubte moche when they here the belles rongen : and this is the cause why the belles ben rongen when it thondreth, and when grete tempeste and outrages of wether happen, to the end that the feindes and wycked spirytes shold be abashed and flee, and cease of the movying of the tempeste." This ringing of the bells of the Church, at the time of thunderstorms, is still practised in many parishes in England.

The God Pan is called in the Orphic Hymns, Jupiter the mover of all things, and is described as harmonising all things by the music of his pipe. (*Hymn. X.*, ver. 12, Fragm. No. xxviii., ver. 13, ed. Gesn.) He is also called the pervader of the sky. (*Orph. Hymn. V.*)

Among the Greeks, all dancing was of the mimetic kind. Dancing was also a part of the ceremonial in all mystic rites, whence it was held amongst the Greeks and Romans in very high esteem. (*Deipnos.*, lib. i., c. xvii.)

Pan is sometimes represented as ready to execute his characteristic office, and sometimes as exhibiting the result of it; in the former, all the muscles of his face and body appear strained and contracted; and in the latter, fallen and dilated; while in both the *phallus* is of disproportionate magnitude, to signify that it represented the predominant attribute. These figures are frequent in collections of small bronzes. The reader, intent on the investigation of these truly (in every view) most important subjects, is confidently referred, for conviction, to the magnificent collection (the choicest and rarest in the world) of Phallic ancient remains from all parts, and gathered from all countries, now deposited in the British Museum.

In one instance, amidst the ancient Phallic objects, Pan appears pouring water upon the instrument (*Bronzi d'Ercolano*, tav. xciii.), but more commonly standing near water, and accompanied by aquatic fowls; in which character he is confounded with Priapus, to whom geese were particularly sacred (*Petronii Satyric*, cxxxvi.—vii.). Hence the Swan of Leda, and his Priapic doings with the heroine, and her enjoyment thereof. Swans frequently occur as emblems of the waters upon coins; and sometimes with the head of Apollo on the reverse. See *Coins of Clazomenæ in Pellerin*, and *Mus. Hunter.*, where may be found some allusion to the ancient notion of their singing; a notion which may have arisen from the noises they make in the high latitudes of the North, prior to their departure, at the approach of winter.

CHAPTER X.

PRIAPIC ILLUSTRATIONS.

ALL students of ancient literature, and the admirers, in the modern day, of the unequalled originality and grace wherewith the Greeks and Romans—particularly the former—invested their ideas, must carefully guard themselves against mingling up their modern prepossessions with the achievements—as they stand before them—of the old-world artists. It is sufficient to reflect that all true art, in its broad sense, comes from the ancients. This art still remains without a rival. Devotional sentiment of quite another order accompanies all the art and literature of the middle ages. The world—and this earthly state for man, so impossible to be understood for its real meaning and ultimate purposes—was treated gloomily. The earth, and the condition of mankind, were regarded as an arena of penitence, of sorrow, of humiliation; and as a condition "lapsed" for some reason, of which man could not see the point, or in reality assent to its justice.

Now, when people began to reflect in the early world upon the vast—the very vast—importance of the sexual relations, which seemed to form the key of all that " was, and is, and is to be"—the tools (to speak the fact strangely)—which were, in their way, to raise, or to build the whole human construction, mind and body ;— these tremendous thoughts as to the " how" in which the whole of this was to be done, impressed and overshadowed, and no wonder that they should so impress and overshadow! The early peoples of the world, finding that Man had already got so much in his own individual personal power, grew to recognise that they had gained a wonderful gift, given to them for some great end, since God had given it. The reflective mind, looking inwards, recognised the Gods—and all the powers of the Gods—in the natural facts of reproduction; the machinery (to use such a word) of which, being so contrary and unexpected, struck them as clearly the result of thought, and of a direct design, not accidental. The objects of this grand display—to speak in the abstract—remained the great puzzle. We think in vastly too light a manner—grown free and presuming in our familiarity—of these truly serious things, now, in the modern day, when science seems to have explained all that is the world.

The Greeks and Romans brought forward the real and the visible—we mean the instruments—of the sexual relations in a way, and with a freedom, inconceivable to those who know nothing of the underlying meaning evident in their gems and coins, and sculpture.

Indeed, so artfully is all this veiled, and so little obvious is the line of connection between the object set forward as an expression, and the thing itself (which is simply in all cases, the conjunction of the sexes), that it requires very considerable practice, and much learning and quick insight, to gather up the meanings. To prove all this, it will be only necessary to refer to the glyptic remains (very remarkable) of which we superadd the descriptions, from a very rare and curious book of the last century, with the title of "Veneres et Priapi." These gems

and coins and fantastic representations come down from
the very remote times of the Rome of the Cæsars.
Priapus, under all his forms, and in his classical, poetical
renderings, whether as Hermes, as Pan, as Faun, as
Shepherd, as single-bodied or as double-bodied, human,
semi-human, half-caprine, block, reversed cone, stone or
stump, bears the same lineaments, the same orbicular
development, the identical metamorphoses and mystic
meaning, and is set up, at all bounds, in innumerable
pillars or posts, or obelisks, or reversed pins, or longitudinal, reversed, pyramidal fragmentary blocks or
shapes, as " God of the Gardens." This strange figure—
Priapus or Pan—with his horns and his hirsute accom-
paniments, with the reeds, and the cymbals, and the
clashes of metal produced in the jar of the

—— " silver-kissing cymbals,"

and the discordant screams and yells and shouts which
accompany him—all of this overpoweringly vehement,
mythic ritual of which the Bacchanals and Bacchantes gave
riotous and disorderly dancing or leaping or convulsionary
expression—is, in certain senses, urged in the world's sense
of things as a protest against the order and regularity of
nature. This Priapus or unnatural grotesque figure may
be treated as a Scarecrow, or as the First of the Scarecrows.
Indecency, according to modern ideas, is pushed to an
extreme in these irregular, lustful scenes. Most of the
representations in " Veneres et Priapi" are too free
(they are all quite the reverse of coarse) to reproduce,
almost to describe. The general impression one bears
away after an examination of these masterpieces of ancient
art, is the false one that the people to whom they were
familiar must have been glaringly sensual and systemati-

cally libidinous. But we must remember that Lycurgus,
who knew nature well, was the first to be convinced that
the free exhibition of the naked human form, whether
male or female, when grown familiar, was the surest
and most complete means of reducing desire within rule
and limit, and of placing irregular eagerness within the
bounds of control. For this reason, that wise and prudent
legislator made it a rule in Sparta that the public gym-
nastic exercises should be partaken of in common by both
males and females. Thus, the races and combats, and
the round of the training for the healthful and beautiful
display of the limbs—of course under proper and judicious
regulations—the games which were always, in their indications and expressions, sacred and mystical, Lycurgus
ordered should be celebrated, in the sight of the whole
of the people, by both youths and maidens in a total
state of nudity. With our modern ideas, this would
seem to be almost impossible. But we can well recognise how all these strange exhibitions, and how all these
most widely accepted Phallic facts, bore sway among the
peoples of antiquity. Every department of the art of the
ancients, in all parts of the world, bears the most unmis-
takable witness of this great truth.

The foregoing observations may be referred more
particularly to the collection of engraved gems, illustrating the remoter mythology of the Greeks and Romans,
published at Leyden some years before the outbreak of
the great French Revolution. This work,* consisting

---

* *Veneres, uti observantur in gemmis antiquis,* Lugd. Batavorum. n.d.
The letterpress in French and English has been attributed to D'Han-
carville, but, we think, he was far too serious an author to express
himself, as he seems to do, with the lightness of the writer of the
preface and notes to this volume.   •

of seventy-one plates, will express things very significant to those who are capable of taking up the meanings of the old, unfortunately discredited theosophy; and, singular in the matter, it is even more remarkable by the manner in which it is presented. The collection may be considered not only as a monumental masterpiece of the fancy of the ancients, but as a memorial of their talents and skill in designing and engraving. "My real opinion," says the author of the preface to the volume, "is that the greatest part of these exceedingly curious engraved stones cannot have been executed before the empire of Augustus and Tiberius." I think it also probable that several of them are the precious figures of Elephantis, the Greek courtesan—which were supposed to be irrecoverably lost, and only surviving in tradition, for their inexpressible success and magnificence in the Venus-like and Priapean sense. This famous Elephantis, not merely the Greek courtesan, but the courtesan *par excellence*, had the audacity (or majestic courage?) to compose books, and to provide illustrations upon the choicest secrets of her profession, in justification and in glory of it.

"Suetonius says that Tiberius had these books placed in his private library, and that the famous 'Aula,' or banqueting-hall in his world-renowned Golden Palace (other historians hint this of Nero) was ornamented with magnificent pictures, painted by the first artists in Rome; pictures twelve in number, and each named after a sign of the zodiac, of life-size, and wholly in the nude; figures displaying the 'twelve postures' in which the Great Act could be the most successfully accomplished—that is, for the purpose of extorting therefrom the most exquisite pleasure, and at the same time of realising the original intentions of Nature in the securing of the most felicitously endowed progeny." Augury, superstition in connexion with those occult studies became, in after ages, in the hands of the adepts, that which was denominated the mystic or celestial anatomy, a framework or mathematical plan of human beings wholly formed in the mysterious invisible regions filled with Rosicrucian Intelligencies, and which was called the "Macrocosm," in contradistinction to that which was styled the "world of man" and his surroundings, or the "Microcosm." All this, in after ages, was demonstrated by the matchless physiologist, Henry Cornelius Agrippa. It formed a mine, a magic mine, worked into by the Rosicrucians, in which all the complexities of astrology, and all the settlements, and the fixing and the poising and the determinatives of the horoscopes of every living human entity born into this world, and all the fatalities of everything, were to be found, caught, as it were, in the eternal web of the necessities of things, as spun by the Immortal Deviser.

The editor of this curious illustrated book thus proceeds:—

"The statement is ascribed to Suetonius that the Emperor Tiberius had some of the designs of the beforementioned superbly accomplished Elephantis placed in certain of his rooms at Capræa, answering the purposes of the volume to which we refer. This voluptuous tyrant is said to have possessed very considerable taste in particular respects.

"*Cubicula plurifariam disposita tabellis, ac sigillis lascivissimarum picturarum, et figurarum adornavit, librisque Elephantidis instruxit.*"

"My intention in publishing this book," adds the editor, "is not in order to save from oblivion the writings of the above-mentioned Elephantis, being persuaded that few will regret such a loss; but as I am certain that the original stones from which I had the designs taken must have been executed by excellent Greek artists, I thought I should not displease the public in reducing them to a form easy to be procured, and which should at the same time show how elegant was the noble simplicity of the ancients, and how far they carried that point of perfection which none of the moderns have yet attained.

"Everybody knows that the most eminent amongst the ancients, such as Zeuxis, Philoxene and Apelles himself, have often amused themselves by painting such kind of subjects: who knows but some of those I am about to produce were of their invention? What I am convinced of is that they could not be better executed."

From the following descriptions of some of the gems (*Veneres et Priapi*) which more closely illustrate our Phallic theme it is hoped that the reader, in the absence of the original work, which is exceedingly rare, may gather a sufficient notion of the freedom with which the ancients celebrated the religious rites of the worship of Priapus:—

Figure IV. represents a sacrifice to the God of the Gardens. The priest who plays upon the double flute is one of those whom Sidonius Apollinaris calls *Mystæ*, because they were equally to serve Priapus and Bacchus. Herodotus calls them *Phalliphori*, or Priapus' carriers, because in processions their business was to carry the symbol of the God of Lampsacus.

Figure XI. Adonis, in the presence of Venus, crowns

the god who is going to give him the preference to Mars.

Festus says that frequently before the young married women were delivered to their husbands they used to be conducted into one of Priapus' temples and made to sit *in sinu ejus.* Figure XII. seems to be a preparation for such a ceremony.

Figure XIII. shows Modesty turning her back on a Priapus concealed in a basket of fruit, which Wantonness presents to her.

Figure XXV. Bacchus and Ariadne prepare themselves to sacrifice to Priapus, in the presence of Love, Satyrs, and Bacchantes.

Figure XXVII. This small figure of brass represents (too obviously for description) Priapus as the god of the gardens.

Figure XXV. In this plate a monster *vulva* stands like a forest tree awaiting the arrival of the emblem of Priapus, which is borne aloft on a triumphal car, with attendant nymphs and cupids.

Figures II. and III. (Part II.) A stone which was formerly in the cabinet of Baron Stock (whose collection the King of Prussia purchased) is engraved on both sides. Messalina, wife of Claudius, is seen sitting before a little chapel in which there is a Priapus; while on the reverse are seven Priapuses surrounding a snail (an animal which, as the naturalists say, having both sexes, is the symbol of lubricity), with the word *Invicta* ("unconquered"), attri-buted to Messalina, and which alludes to that verse of Juvenal, *Et lassata viris nondum satiata recessit.*

Figure V. is a terminal of Priapus, with the attribute of Hercules, in order to commemorate the exploit of the god in connexion with the forty-nine daughters of Thespius, King of Bœotia.

Figure VI. represents a dialogue between a "very magnificent Priapus" and a man who puts his ear to it, as if waiting for an answer, in supposed allusion to the violence of passion which speaks with such energy that nothing else is heard.

Figure VII. shows a kind of wheel of a lottery, the prizes attached to which are emblems of Priapus. Cupid turns the wheel with difficulty, a female on each side seeming to retard its progression.

Figure VIII. A terminal of Priapus with the Thyrsus of Bacchus, which alludes to Horace's verse, *Sine Cerere et Baccho friget Venus*.

Figure XI. A Satyr riding upon a Priapus.

Figure XV. A Bacchante, with her knees upon a basket, consecrates a small figure to Priapus, while another woman sitting in a basket plays upon the double flute. The mysterious basket shows that this god's operations ought to be secret.

Figure XVII. The usual divinity, easily recognised by his natural figure, is walking upon a cock's legs. Compare with XXV.

Figure XXIII. A young hero sacrificing to Priapus. On the top of the column, upon which the emblem of the god is engraved, is a lighted fire.

Figure XXV. A cupid riding upon a Priapus, with a lion's legs, holds the bridle and a whip, to show how Love is able to tame Passion.

Figure XXVI. Ceremonies performed at the feast of Priapus. The god, standing upon a column, is surrounded with branches of the olive-tree, either because he is the protector of the gardens or because he loves peace, of which the olive-tree is the symbol.

Figure XXVII. Venus, followed by a young man, presents to Priapus some branches of myrtle. Behind the terminal of the god (who is represented under the figure of a young man in the vigour of his age) a Satyr plays upon the flute and dances. In the meantime Love burns his bow upon the altar, which is adorned with wreaths, as on a festival.

Figures XXX. and XXXI. Two Priapuses of an immoderate size found in the environs of Albano, the ancient Alba.

Figure XXXIV. A nude female performs a sacrifice to Priapus by pouring wine upon the flames which issue from a brazier at the foot of his statue.

The denomination of Mercury as the god of the frontiers, the borders or limits among the Germans and the Celts, was applied to all the mark-stones, or stones of the boundaries, which indicated the confines of any particular domain. This application, together with the sacred ideas which always went with these monuments, was introduced into that part of Italy to which the Romans gave the name of Cisalpine Gaul, by the Celts or Gauls who effected the conquest of the country, and established in it their usages and religion. Through this introduction Italy came to possess two separate divinities, though both were in certain respects identical in character. Two different names were ascribed to them in regard to an inflection or a change of their potentiality. With one meaning they were called Termes, or the Terminals, or the "fixed." With another they were called the "varying." France furnishes a great number of names indicative of the worship of

Mercury. The monolithic monuments all owe their destination to the same ideas. In innumerable forms, whether
the form be slender, as the terminal raised in honour of
Pan, or of Mercury, the God of Boundaries (the veritable
Priapus); or whether the forms be columns of large
size, or stones, hewn and sculptured, either bulky or
rough, whether called Thoths, Hermes, Bethels, Bethyles,
Menhirs, or by whatever name they were denominated,
they all, in various mystic forms and in far-off references,
assume the PHALLIC meaning as the all-important hint.
In ancient times, by a sort of sublime general signal as
tracing to a certain centre-point of abstract particular
significance, these votive objects covered the earth. They
were the most distinctly and frequently to be met with,
and they were the more enlivened (so to express the
idea) in their vividness of expression and in their astute
direct address (in their meaning to the spectator) in proportion to the extent to which art had become expansive
and imaginative; but the idea flourished in some form in
all the countries of which there are monuments and in
which civilisation and poetry and philosophy most successfully throve.

The worship of the Phallus was greatly cultivated
among the Gauls. It does not appear that much attention this way, or as afforded to this worship, became
conspicuous anterior to the arrival of the Romans. Logs,
pieces of wood, and longitudinal stems were fixed up to
represent, sometimes, these figures as presiding over boundaries. The ancients placed on the summit of these
significant figures a human head, and, in continuation, a
part of a masculine body. Thus erected and detailed in
whole, or, more commonly, in part, these " bounds," or

terminals, or blocks of wood, or trunks of trees, constituted the Hermes, the Termes, the Mercuries, or those
idols or halves of men, that our artists have reproduced
in so many classic forms, most of which are very beautiful.
In course of time the origin of these diverse figures, thus
metamorphosed, thus strangely composed, grew indistinct
in the ideas of the peoples. The Phallus idol with the
feet of the goat, placed in the fields or erect in the midst
of cultivated lands, became the god Pan. Placed in the
groves, in the forests, or amidst the mountains, it was the
Faun, the Silvan, the Satyr. Amongst the vines the
figure saluted the observer as Bacchus. At the limits of
territories, in the public ways, at cross-roads, or at the
entrances of villas or dwelling-houses, the Idol Phallus
received the name of Hermes Casmillus, or Mercury, with
the distinguishing masculine points openly displayed or
more covertly or slyly suggested, according to the freedom of the ideas prevailing in the district.

We will terminate this section of our history with the
following interesting particulars, drawn from the " Divinités Génératrices chez les Anciens et les Modernes"
of J. A. Dulaure. At page 417 of the second volume
of the second edition the author says :—

" Les vases" (a case collateral with all the classic vases)
"dont je viens d'indiquer les peintures lascives étaient
des objets religieux. Ils sont dans le Musée du Roi de
Naples, à Capo di Monte. Ils ont été decouverts dans
des tombeaux, près de Nola ; et l'on sait que les tombeaux étaient, chez les anciens, sacrés comme le sanctuaire.

" Le savant auteur qui a décrit ces vases, et publié les
dessins de leur peinture, vient à l'appui de mon opinion.
' On rencontre,' dit il, ' dans les monuments, une mul-

titude de *Priapées*; on en trouve même dans les lieux
les moins susceptibles de les recevoir: ce qui prouve
combien les Grecs étaient familiarisés avec ces images que,
dans nos mœurs, nous nommons obscènes.

"'Les *Priapées*, représentées comme objets religieux,
sont en très-grand nombre—Quelque système qu'on
se fasse à cet égard, il faut toujours revenir à cette idée
principale, que les anciens n'y voyaient qu'un emblème
de la nature fécondante, et de la reproduction des êtres
qui servent à la composition et à l'entretien de l'univers.
C'est à cette idée que nous devons ces Priapes de toutes
les formes qu'on rencontre dans les cabinets, et ces
offrandes de toute espèce, qui rappellent le culte du dieu
de Lampsaque.'

"Le même auteur parle de lampes antiques qui offrent
des images licencieuses, et dont plusieurs sont conservées
à la Bibliothèque Royale : il croit qu'elles pouvaient être
appliquées à l'usage de la religion.

"Il cite les pierres gravées, et même ces médailles,
appelées *spintriennes*, qui représentent, à ce que l'on a
cru, les débauches de Tibère dans l'île de Caprée, et les
bizarres accouplemens auxquels il donnait le nom de
Spintriæ. Il place au rang des plus célèbres productions
antiques de ce genre le groupe du Satyre et la chèvre
du Musée de *Portici*, qu'on ne peut voir qu'avec une
permission particulière ; un autre groupe, à peu près
semblable, trouvé à Nettuno, vendu par le cardinal
Alexandre Albani au dernier roi de Pologne, et conservé
actuellement à Dresde ; le Priape du Musée du cardinal
Albani, avec 'l'inscription,' et le Priape du Musée de
Florence.

"Si l'on s'étonnait moins de ce que la religion des

anciens a commandé des sacrifices humains, le plus grand attentat contre les sociétés, que de ce qu'elle a consacré l'acte de la reproduction des êtres, acte conservateur de l'espèce humaine ; s'il nous paraissait moins étrange de voir l'homme abuser, par piété, de son penchant à la cruauté que de le voir abuser, par le même motif, de sa propension naturelle aux plaisirs de l'amour, nous ferions nous-mêmes la satire de nos propres opinions, et nous avouerions notre préférence pour un culte qui détruit et donne la mort à celui qui conserve et donne la vie."

CHAPTER XI.

TRANSCENDENTAL IDEAS OF THE ROSICRUCIANS. THEIR CABALISTIC PHILOSOPHY AS TO THE OCCULT INTERCHANGE OF NATURE, AND OF MAGIC.

FROM a considerable amount of the foregoing matter, in this Book, there may arise, in the unprepared reader's mind, a feeling, first of surprise, and then of dissent—although we do not think that this sensation of dissent will degenerate—certainly not upon second thoughts—into displeasure. We have introduced particulars of truths; and have grouped truths round about particulars; but in no case have we written except after very deep and doubtful and (we may securely add) very suspicious and rigorous examination. However questionable, however out-of-the-way, and however heterodox, our comment may sometimes appear to shallowly-judging persons, we hope to be generally criticised coolly and sagaciously. Most modern opinion is class opinion,—is narrow-minded opinion; in fact, no opinion whatever. We protest, beforehand, against the assumptions of these classes; who *seem* to stand upon good presupposed grounds, and to exercise authority, in regard to these peculiar subjects; but who, in reality, do neither. We wish to be judged, in these undoubtedly singular, and seemingly defiantly eccentric, forthcoming passages, with more magnanimity and large-mindedness than we consider prevails with most modern critics. We are aware that we stand very independently (although it is some comfort to know that we have the ancients with us) in the views which we entertain upon these mysterious and all-important sexual and theosophical subjects. But we wish to be understood as universally deprecating hasty judgment upon them. The opinion which "comes uppermost" is generally wrong, not only upon these topics, but not infrequently upon *all* topics in respect of which there may be inquiry. We desire to bespeak a free arena for all our ideas—and they are, in far-prevailing preponderance, explanatory in one way or other of the notions of that renowned, and yet carefully and essentially mysterious succession of men, the much-debated Rosicrucians. The " R. C." sought resolutely to stand aloof from all mankind, in certain very peculiar respects. They were determined to trample upon the base parts of their nature—to turn from the temptation and to refuse the embraces of women. And yet the object of their adoration was the " Rose," thence one of their names and the one half of their distinguishing title—the " Rose," with all the mystical meanings, which, as it were impersonated, follow with the ideas of that flower—the " Queen" of the " Garden," most glorious when renewed, and recalled to life, in the " shower." The " Brothers of the R. C." were, also, ordained to poverty, yet set aside, as Saints, to effect all the good they could in the world—themselves remaining unseen, unknown, and unhonoured; considered as possessing all the riches of the world in their secret, supernatural powers over the invisible world as the " rulers of the spirits;" the means of the perpetuation of youth and beauty; all gifts, divine and human, as the " Sons of God," and access to the councils of the angels and archangels—yet bearing the Cross of Christ, and only glorified in the sufferings, and in the sacrifice of the

Immortal Redeemer, who Himself, although the Son of God, took upon himself all the sins and imperfections of humanity, and submitted to become a servant, and at last to be despised and mocked, and affixed, with the piercing nails (metaphorically and mystically, as Jacob Behmen says, " struck through both worlds" of the " visible" and the " invisible"), upon the accursed "Tree !"

In all matters brought forward in this Book, and duly (and certainly cautiously) placed before our readers in our successive Chapters, we fall back (quietly, though with confidence,) upon conclusions which have been only arrived at—after much pausing—even *suspicious* pausing— at the successive stages of acquirement.

However bold and audacious the theory may appear to rose-water philosophers, and to sentimentalists of a certain order, we will lay the moral, and the reasons for the moral, before the reader in a few words. This theory pre-assumes, in the abstruse sense, that there is no virtue so pure, lofty, and genuine, as that virtue which yields and surrenders when there is no escape for it :—resigning simply *when it can do no more;* when all means of resistance are exhausted ; when *force* (which is the key to unlock the submission of all the worlds, bodily and spiritual) is *master.* The unfortunate Lucretia—though her self-sacrifice sprang from a most noble soul—there-fore (in this view) made a mistake in dying, instead of living. Force, which is the master of the world, was present in the form of her ravisher. He might even have acknowledged the authority of the gods, and justified himself—nay, applauded himself—by the example of all the gods. This philosophic view of the case has never yet been admitted, simply because the world has fallen

into a sudden passion of indignation at Tarquin's act. It
will, here, at once be seen that it was Christianity alone—
or the idea of Christianity—which gave to the world that
sublime character, the "Knight-Errant," and realised all
the grand system of championship, pervading throughout,
and prevailing in the feudal system, and its perfect chain
of obligations and honours, reaching in unbroken corresponding and complementary succession from the crown—
truly even down to the sense of duty, and of gratitude in
the serf, who worked for his own sustainment, protected
by his lord, and submissive to the ruling of God. It
was only in the abuses of these great and good things
that rapine, violence, robbery, and wrong arose. But to
pass to our argument. Combating for that which is
called sexual virtue to the "bitter-end," or to the last, is a
mistake and an error of outrage against oneself and of
foolhardiness; a misrendering of true conduct, even in
the cause of the most exalted virtue itself. Hence—however fine and grand in theory—and doubtless so far as
the individuality, or the person himself, or herself (the
female, particularly) is concerned, it is grand—the folly of
such gratuitous heroism—which is surely "self-murder"
if anything be—is clear. This condition of inviolability
of the body (mechanism, however exquisite), in face of the
very character and nature of the body, which was formed
for the enjoyment, in perfection, of the very Act which is
thus petulantly and obstinately flung back in the face of
the very contriver of it all—which is known as Nature—
is, after all, unnatural.

Why should arise this misplaced enthusiasm—this
blind, gratuitous defence—this clinging to the idea of the
fighting to the last for the citadel which it is the very

intention of Nature to throw open to the occupation? Why this destruction of self in this self-assumed supposed defence of spotlessness and virginity when everything depends upon the infraction thereof? There is accepted a universal conviction which all the persuasions of common sense cannot remove, or obliterate, or charm to sleep, or even compel to suspension, that all this rigid, unbargaining defence of virtue means glory and holiness. From this—the saints in heaven! from this—the protests to the all-judging gods—the gods of all time and of all place, who are only to be known by the possibility of a human consciousness or conscience, and therefore only by man (as produced by woman). Nature itself knows nothing of this contradictory appeal. To Nature it is *rebellion*, for it is the first thing ordained of Nature, and Nature is fullest of contrivances for its plenitude of indulgence. In the face of these truths, in the acknowledgment of all philosophy, in the redemption of the civilised times from the onrush of barbarism, and the lowering of the sublimest artistic instincts peopling the world of mind and of matter with beauties, the office of the woman in serving *this* purpose stands exalted as the most transcendent proof of the intentions of the gods in regard of her and of her exalted honour and beneficence in the carrying out of the resolutions of the councils of the world's makers. Instead of there being, properly, shame and disgrace in the application of herself to the satisfaction of these instincts, and in the fulfilling of her destiny to the end of the free life, and of the free companionship (always in the abstruse sense), when we examine into the realities of things, instead of degradation there is admiration. It is from these reasons that, among the ancients, the very name of " harlot"* was abstractedly

* Mr. Myles McSweeney, in a letter to the author dated April 4th,
1871, says :—" The word (an important word) 'Al' in Arabic stands
for the 'Uza,' Venus—*i.e.*, the 'Woman.' I submit the term 'Venus'
is derived from the Chaldaic 'Benoth' (Women). The Greeks changed
the B to V and the terminal 'oth' to 'os,' hence 'Ven*os*,' or, as we
have the word from the Latins, 'Ven*us*.' There is no doubt but that
the Arabic 'Uza' is derived from the Hebrew 'Aishe, the Woman,'
or, as the Greeks call her, 'Isis.' Venus, we know, had two characters.   There were two ways of regarding the 'Female' in the old
world, and this distinction is maintained through the whole mythology
of the Greeks, and therefore, of course, through the whole of the mythology, or the history of the Court of Olympus and of the doings of the
gods of the Romans, who adopted and altered (not for the better)
the religious ideas and the supereminently beautiful fables of the Greeks.
'Venus,' or 'Isis,' or the 'Woman,' or the 'Goddess' of all the ancient
religions, 'shone' (or 'displayed'?) through the myths in two characters
—bad and good; and these characters were continuously interchanging,
or, in other words, they were (mystically, of course,) *identical*. There
was the chaste Venus, or, using other expressions, the triumphant, sacred
'Virgin,' who shared the characteristics of the unconquered and the
invincible Diana, who, when seen in her nakedness, and therefore in
her profanation, was cited as a sacred personage with the office of
launching the magic penalty by the power of transfixing with the curse,
which terror and annihilation (as Man) Diana inflicts on Actæon, who
was, in consequence, torn to pieces by the avenging demons in the
shape of his own hounds.   The chaste Venus—if the idea of Venus is
ever that of chastity—was the 'Venus Urania,' or the Venus of the
stars, or of heaven. The 'Venus Pandemos' was the harlot. I am
fully convinced, as a result of the most careful consideration of all these
purposely confused and incessantly (designedly) evading matters, that
from this Arabic word 'Uza' we derive the word 'Hussey,' as applied
to ladies who let themselves out to hire or who feel disposed to worship
this Venus Pandemos in their own particular—very acceptable, doubtless—manner.   Hence our word 'whore' (see Bailey)—*i.e.*, 'hired
women for prostitution.' The word 'hire' in Hebrew is 'Shaker.'
We know the 'G' and 'K' are interchangeable letters, hence 'Shagger.'
Whether these coincidences are only accidental or not it is not very
easy to declare, but, nevertheless, the fact is very curious, and it seems
to prove a good deal that they so closely correspond to each other."

esteemed sacred, and the profession looked upon not only as necessary but as grand and praiseworthy. The dignity and defiance (as it were, in the noble sense,) of the infraction of virtue was held great under certain circumstances. The interest and the respect was always the sublimest, the reader may remark, in the cases of enforced violation. The sustainment of this kind of life, from necessity, was honoured by the State, and was surrounded by a peculiar sort of sanctification. Hence, in certain aspects, and arising from certain considerations, the stupendous dignity and holiness of the "Magdalen" —she the mysterious idea of whom (in the occult sense) was commensurate with the trembling of Heaven, of Earth, and of the last member of the "Eternal Triplicate"—the Nether Regions—knowing of dole, knowing of "Fire," knowing of the "punishments" for the "Presumption," which is hinted, in the "Cabala," as the cause of having emptied Heaven of "One Third" of its Inhabitants, consequently realising the "Second Fall," that in which the Human Race is concerned, or the "Fall of Man," necessitating religion, bringing about, through the Divine Benignity, the offered "Redeemer," or the Propitiatory Christ, to insure the change in the "Divine Intentions," which secured everything, according to the Cabalists.*

---

* Those were indeed bold explorers into the wonders of the natural world. Salt and fire have properties in common. Salt, like a subtle fluid, penetrates all that is corruptible and separates that which is decaying and foul, whilst it quickens that which is sound. Fire destroys that which is perishable, and thereby establishes the imperishable in its purest perfection, and leads to new and more beautiful forms of being. Thus both effect a kind of transformation. Now 'Every one, our Lord saith, shall be salted with fire,' by his being involuntarily salted with the fire

But to pass back to our singular theme in regard to the prevalent though natural error in the consideration of that feeling called female virtue, of course only in the abstract and in the philosophical and transcendental sense. We do not wish to consider this strange and mysterious subject in any other light—we mean from any other point of view—than the philosophical and the merely controversial and speculative. Let us reflect for a few moments upon the important part which the "Idea" of the "Magdalen" plays in the results and in the philosophical conclusions of the whole round of the universal Theosophy. It lies *perdu* side by side with the sacred mysticism accompanying the theological reveries or dreams—true, as all dreams in the lesser or the larger extension are "true enough," although truly so only "in their own world," which is the world of the mysteries, which again surround and make a mere island, as it were, of the real and the true—according to "man's truth," truth that, in reality, out of the commonplace reality—to use a paradox—"is no truth at all." The idea of the Magdalen is that of the twin sister of Virginity: of the other sister (or twin sister), or the "White Sister" to this "Red Sister" ("red with sin"). In this occult and Gnostic sense she is the Glorious Counterpart, or "Sister," as a transformed, holiest mystic means, of the "Sacred Virgin"—the Virgin Mary herself—the Miraculous Heroine, star-crowned "lily-invested," of the "Annunciation"—proclaimed by the "Chiefest Friend to Man among the Archangels," the Angel Gabriel, the

of condemning judgment (Heb. x. 27, xii. 29), as the victims on the altar were salted with salt (Levit. ii. 13, Ezek. xliii. 24. See Lange).

*Cab-*ala itself, as is seen by a little reflection. " C" and
" G" mean the same thing in all languages, in all their
marks or symbols or hieroglyphics.

Thus we arrive at certain mystic conclusions, or "arch-
conclusions." Hence, in certain ways, the stupendous
dignity and holiness of " The Magdalen"—she out of
whom, as the " Woman-Conqueror" after all—the
" female Saint Michael"—were cast "seven devils." She—
this sainted, this deified " Being"—be it ever remembered,
was "first" at the Tomb of the Redeemer. The mysticism of this impressive side of Christianity is the most
beautiful in the world. All this view is exhibited most
powerfully in the writings of the great mystic, Jacob
Behmen. Necessity makes the glory of the loss of
virginity, or the supernatural dignity, in the heroic sense,
of enforced prostitution. Martyrdom is a mistake in this
reading of obligations. For Death in Escape—we are
not all martyrs, nor can we be such, nor is it intended by
Nature that we be such—Death in Escape, we repeat,
is not only the bitterest but it is the *mistaken* door out of
which to fly. There is no virtue so perfectly beautiful,
however paradoxical it may seem, as that Virtue which is
forced into submission in the *instant's necessity*, with its
protest and appeal, when Heaven turns away its head,
and, obdurate as the rock to the shriek, *seems* as if it
would not hear !

> " Is there no pity, sitting in the clouds,
>   To see into the bottom of my grief ?"

Thus Juliet cries in her despair. The outraged one, with
the barbarous hands of Hell's force upon her, figuratively,
as it may be said—and it is no irreverence to say so, since
it occurs as obvious—seems, in that cry of vain despair,

to fling back, protesting, the outrage—to speak vividly—
indignantly, from "this side Nature," into the very lap of
the gods that permit it,—those very gods, here assumed
as the incontestable Divinity, who make and ordain the
sacrifice—that destruction to which the Victim succumbs.
Ay, the virtue which is prostituted over the face of the
whole earth is never in reality touched! Talk not to us
of escapes! *The world has no escapes.* Least of all are
there escapes in death.

CHAPTER XII.

CONSIDERATIONS ON THE MYSTIC ANATOMY OF THE ROSICRUCIAN PHILOSOPHERS.

THE heroes of the Holy Graël are the divine guardians of its meanings. They are chosen of God, set aside in their purity, and although gifted with the might of Mars, or the valour and address and the sublime angelic strength of the shepherd-boy David, they are harmless to all the humble, deserving, and good, and are the chosen exe-cutants of the heavenly purposes, to be committed alone to those " spotless as children." In a sense, partly (when adopted into the higher forms of God's service, which service assumes all sorts of ranks and degrees, and all forms of superiority, and of inferiority, in the ascending, according to the gifts and movements upward of the server, or of the heavenly-assisted influences—the more effectually or the less effectually availed of),—the cham-pions of the Holy Graël were gradually cleared of their mortal disabling conditions. They progressed, according to their purity, in magic power. They acquired beauty upon beauty and grace upon grace, kindled in new know-ledge, passed up into a newer level of excellence, and acquired, when they were accepted, the mysterious double nature, the possibility of which is known only in the counsels of the Almighty, by which, when despatched to discharge some particular office of championship as the servant-soldiers of the Lord, they resigned, temporarily, their semi-angel character and passed to earth as men, and mixed in the affairs of men, and lived and mingled with people in the ordinary way with a man's body, only to be glorified and to be testified to (in the assurance of all) transitorily, as more than human when they chose to display themselves as superhuman. Thus from the tale of the champion Lohengrin we learn that the warrior is the sacred mystic brother of the undiscoverable monastery, or hold, or fortress, or castle, or hermitage, or palace—whatever name we choose to give it—of the mysterious Mount of Safety, or Salvation, or " *Mont Salvagge*," or " *Selvaggio*," that " castled peak" amidst the encircling woods, which, although sought for ever by human foot and eye, is never to be found except through the assent of the brothers themselves. The knight is represented as rising from his knees there in the " Chapel of the Graël," before the altar of which he passes his days and nights in ceaseless prostrate adoration. He hears the single warning quiet stroke of the holy bell, which declares that in some part of the world (as yet unknown) some deserving sufferer groans or shrieks in " sore strait," and that he (the champion) is the one selected and summoned for the surpassing duty of the interference and the rescue. Armed and helmed, with his mailed foot ready to be placed in his knightly stirrup, and his hand twisted in the long mane of his charger, ready to mount, the champion, with his eyes raised to heaven in expectation, waits for the magic sign which shall convey to him its hieroglyphical directions. The orders arrive; the path is pointed out. He resigns himself to invisible guidance. In his dream, or in his sleep,—couchant like the glorious lily flower upon his burnished shield which flashes to the light his cognizance, the " silver swan,"—the knight Lohengrin fancies that he is traversing the latitudes "a thousand miles or more, or many more." He thus proceeds until, to the last summons of the trumpets of the heralds, and in almost the despair of the masses of the people, all gathered to witness the destruction, doubtless by the fire or severing sword, of the fated Princess Elsa of Brabant, the approaching boat, towed by something which seems to the people like a magnificent swan, impossible for its size, its whiteness and beauty, nears the strand. The wondrous Knight of the Graël—the holy saint or angel Lohengrin—treads to the shore, welcomed by the shouts of the Flemish multitude, awestruck in the miracle of the sight, but intoxicated with joy. It is a sudden and a signal rescue. How the champion sped, how he fought, how he conquered, how he lived among the people familiarly for his prescribed period, how he was honoured by being raised to the highest rank by the emperor, Henry the Fowler, "Enrico Uccelerato," how the rescued Elsa fell in mad, passionate love with her deliverer (as how could she help it or withstand such wondrous gifts?), how Lohengrin reciprocated her love as far as he could or dared, consistently with the awful vows of resignation and of abnegation which avow him as one of the elect holy knights of the "Graël," sworn to denial of and impossibility of approach by the embraces of woman; how the wail or plaint of the "sacrifice" implied in the feigned marriage is sung as a dirge* to the intertwining mazes

* Of course the people of the Principality of Brabant do not know of the real character of this pretended, ill-starred, impossible marriage with their princess, for the apparent human knight Lohengrin is taken by the concourse for a real man, as also by the bride and the emperor and his court. He is only suspected for his real character by

of the solemn wedding-dance, so significant of German mysticism, and termed the " Torch-Dance of the Bridal," or the famous Fackeltanz, almost always performed at court and other grand weddings, which in such a serious country as Germany are solemnities ; how all these stirring and weird and strangely-interesting circumstances and events came to pass, and what is their (even historical) issue we shall leave the historians of the Teutonic profundities to declare, and the romancists of the German Fatherland more fully to describe and to embellish. Further, let the profound musical intricacies and the deep-dreaming of the sometimes over-clouded meanings and purposes of the

the enchantress Ortrud and by the evil-minded intending assassin Telramond when he is vanquished. The Knights of the Graël were bound never to reveal their real character, and to forsake all their human engagements and entanglements at the first recall to their secret habitation or castle. The council of the Knights or Brothers of the Holy Grail, or Graël, was a reflex of the sacred bond sanctified by sacraments which held the majestic and mystic Rosicrucians together. These were really the guardians of the greater mysteries. In this sense of the mysterious and the sacred, the "garter" of the "Most Noble the Order of the ' Garter' "—the first of chivalry—is not a " garter" at all, but the "*Garder*," or " Keeper," the sacredest and holiest guardian of the supernatural chastity of none other than the most exalted feminine personality (of course in the abstract and miraculous sense), the very foundation of Christianity—the "Cestus" or girdle of the blessed and immaculate Virgin Mary, the Queen of Heaven, with her victorious foot, for all the ages past and to come, trampling upon the Dragon, in her celestial purity, as the "Mother of Christ."

In advancing this very original and unexpected but genuine reading of the mysteries which appertain subjectively to this magnificent order, we can at once see the absurdity of conferring the order upon sovereigns or princes or upon any persons who are not Christians, however politically important they may seem to the people of England. Heralds and skilled archæologists and philosophers, who are presumed to be people of penetration, will perceive all this at once.

composer Wagner be had recourse to in order to raise the mind and attune the interest and attention to the meta-physical subtleties involved in the adequate consideration of the design, authority, and weight of this legend, or story, or fable, or history, or allegory (or truth, to a certain impressive extent), of Lohengrin, the Knight of the Sangrael, at once the puzzle of all commentators, of all antiquaries, nay, of all Christianity. But, understood or not, the whole story is very beautiful, poetically graphic and interesting, and at the same time religious and sacred.

In brief, and as an explanation of their supposed real character, the knights of King Arthur's court were aim-ing to achieve, by their efforts in this world and in their acts of rescue and of beneficence, their presumed angel-assisted traverse up the difficult heights set with moral precipices to the aspiring heaven.

They were, in their worldly character as holy pilgrims, set a task, sworn to sacred obligations, united in a fraternity whose distinguishing mark and boast were the maintenance among themselves of rites and of an elaborate knightly—even monastic—rule as nearly as possible and as far as was consistent with the continual necessary exercise of their warlike calling. They were enjoined to this so long as their youth and powers and the spirit of adventure remained to inspire them with the uses of the elaborate cere-monial. These masters in the profession of chivalry realised the active and sublime knightly characteristics in the old days, ages before the false idea entered men's minds that their *only* purpose in the world was to engage in commerce and in buying and selling and exchanging and bargaining, in adding this item to that item, in con-solidating the increase, and in realising capital. The capital they sought was the accumulation of health, of peace and quietness, of comfort and happiness, of rest, enjoyment, and competence. Their aims were moderate wants and satisfaction, knowledge and wisdom, piety, and hope, and trust. Compare this unworldly life, and the ideas that these heroes entertained of the enchantments of music,* with

* The ideas of the ancients as to the character and the power of music were very remarkable. The music of the spheres was the grand harmonious rhapsody—the life and breath and language of the divinities, wherewith the gods first imagined, and then "built up" and "endowed" Nature. Thus music is magical, and we have in it the tradition of the first state, or of Paradise, now feebly, intermittently recalled as hints —that are so sad that they move to tears as in a " dream."

The Rosicrucians contend that music, or melody, which is enchantment, pervades all nature in its prosperous or intended progress, although it is only the wail, or plaint, of the instinctive soul on its wounded, or sacrificed, or " Ruined" Side. It mourns for its Original Lost Paradise. The music of the spheres is no unreal thing, but real as is the atmosphere of the spirits. For music is as the atmosphere of the spirits and discords, though the necessary support and balance of Creation, are a medium for the coarse and low spirits, who inundate, as it were, the lees and settlings of Nature, or the shadows and dark places of Nature ; for the *bass* is as necessary to emphasise and to bring out and support the lighter, or motived side of music, as the shadows are indispensable to supply the life and reality to objects in the real world. It is only the responsive soul of man that is moved by music. The lower animals have no sense of music, although there is no doubt that they have a means of communicating with each other, or some sort of language. But the lower animals are all stopped short at something (whatever it be, for it is totally unknown by man), which state has the effect as of a sort of limited dream to them, and therefore they make no progress, although they have certain spiritual perceptions greater and more delicate than mankind. The whole world is taken as a musical instrument. Heavenly music is produced from melodious supernatural impact upon the paths of the planets, which stand, as chords or strings, by the cross-travel of the sun, in the ecliptic, from star to star, and from note to note, or from planet to planet. Earthly music is microscopically an imitation of the same, and a relic of heaven. The Rosicrucians taught that all nature is the mean pursuits of the moderns, wholly given over to common things. These mystical persuasions, abounding in that remote early time when religious feeling was possible, when reverence and respect for sacred ideas and theosophical theses were possible, when the modes and methods of life were either markedly simple or grandly and impressively magnificent, when poverty was only comparative on account of the fewness of wants, and the curse of conceit and of pride was neither so prevalent nor so fierce nor so flagrant. These fearing doubts, this emphasising and humanising into forms and voices of the forces of Nature, and this solicitous invoking or assuagement of the friendliness, or the hostilities, of the outside powers into accessible personality, into concentrate motived end, into intelligence, into spite and persecution, or assistance and guardianship and defence, all placed under special rule and committed to the charge of subordinated invisible spirits or ministers, benevolent or malign or neutral, actors or witnesses or both; call all this superstition, and say that these romantic, highly-toned fervid motions were mere delusion and dreaming, the result of a state of society unintelligible to the moderns. Granting all this—nay, conceding more :—and how far are we advanced in the conviction of the true certainty of our gains, and of the meaning and purport of the march of the

produced, like a piece of music, by melodious combinations of the cross movement of the holy light playing over the lines of the planets, light flaming as the spiritual ecliptic, or the *gladius* of the Archangel Michael, to the frontiers or extremities of the solar system. "Music, colours, and language (the vowels of the latter intermittent through the mouth, and therefore producing speech), the *phenomena* (in the world) of music, colours, and language are allied."—"*The Analogy of the Laws of Musical Temperament to the Natural Dissonance of Creation,*" by M. Vernon. London: 1867. See also "The Rosicrucians," p. 235 *et supra.*

generations? We think that the story of the centuries tells in reality of no progress. The world revolves in a never-ending circle. Civilisations rise and fall, contradict each other, change wholly in their character. But that is all. Nations only advance to achieve their highest point, and then to recede. Such is the fate of communities, such the fate of individuals, such is the fate of the world.

CHAPTER XIII.

ROSICRUCIAN PROFUNDITIES.

IT is an assertion of the occult philosophers that the meaning and purpose of life is altogether mistaken. That is—that it is necessarily—in the "necessity of things"—mistaken. That, inasmuch as *he lives*, man is incapacitated for pronouncing upon the *nature of his life;* being it—*itself.* He being a "liver" is "it"—(*i.e.,* "life, itself.") These positions are obvious, when thus stated. Philosophy and common sense take it for granted that life needs consciousness, or some form in which the consciousness may reside, in order that the liver may "live." Abstract philosophy asserts that the liver (living) unlives (in the true sense) *for the very purpose of living.* In other words, it is concluded that, as man is the "thing seen," the individual cannot ever go out of himself, "to see himself." The "judged at the bar" cannot cease his character to become another character, and to change places with his judge, and become the judge on the bench. The individual cannot go out of "himself" to become "something other than himself" and to judge of what he is, himself.

Now all this, obviously, cannot be in common sense, or in any sense. And, in this manner, this philosophy is applied in the Hermetic sense. The alchemists contended that it is possible (by art) to obtain out of the boundless, holy, unappropriated eternal youth of Nature, a wherewithal by means of which to "wreak"—to use a strange

word. Thus there could be miraculous renewal possible
even out of the existent powers of Nature.

No one knows the purposes of God, nor can any one
limit the powers of God. No one can apply the word
" impossible" to the powers of God Almighty; for the
word " possible" only applies to man's (false) notions of
things, which apprehension only springs from his senses;
which culminate, in the sum and perfection of all his
senses, in his reason; and his senses do not make reason,
for they rather make *unreason.* Farther, we will state
the case still more strongly (if more curiously) when we
say that it is the real fact, in the one sense (the abstract
sense) that men only " die," because they do not " live
any longer;" because that " which lives in them" cannot
any longer maintain itself in them. It is not the man,
but the thing that is *in* the man, that dies. Thus men
really (and only) die by the very means by which they
live—that is, by the natural nutriment or the means of
destruction (however slow) by which they live. Very
naturally fire should cease to burn itself out, in the con-
sumption and decomposition and using up of the fuel by
which the fire (the life in the world of elements) is produced and maintained. The natural nutriment is the
indefinitely-delayed corrosion, the slow means of destruction. Digestion is destroying agitation, in the body, of
its kind; which, in time, wears out the solids, and brings
on decrepitude. All the phenomena of this—as it were—
eating away or natural nutrition, is as the flameless fire
which feeds upon the solids, and at last consumes man.
The true art to live is to eat as little as possible, to
maintain the body in its balance of health. And as to
decease, man dies daily in his bodily secretions, and

therefore corruptions. In the abstract sense, *he is always dying*, because digestion is natural corruption, and corruption is digestion, or disintegration, or dissolution, as we have before said. This gift of death in life is the NATURAL result of mortality—is the only condition by means of which we live. Food is as fuel, which, in its working up, and in its elaboration, just as truly destroys, just as flame destroys, only in a non-inflammable manner. The Hermetical philosophers held that it is possible to arrest, in magic art, the supernatural secret seeds (operative though invisible) of new life in the next world, off this world, which was certainly not all spirit. They held to a peculiar opinion that particular life is only an arrest out of the broad flow of general life; the quicker, the slower, in its effervescence of fructification (as growing plants) as it became the more quickly purged of the thicker matter, and as the divine motived spark set itself forward the speedier and surer, as the freer out of its coagulation, choke, or devil-like and impeding hindrances. We know how short the minutest microscope goes of reality. Man's registers and instruments fail him above and below. Thus his science only commands a part—and a very limited part—of the real. A continual assertion of the Rosicrucians is, that the philosopher's fire is to be found in everything ; that the *germen* of the *lapis philosophorum* abides in everything. But that the elimination of this unknown, inside matter, or ensouled magnetism, or spirit of Nature, or means of endowment, in possibility of renewable life (in the interior of all life, motived and spiritual) is their own affair, and that the secret of attaining to it rests solely and wholly in their hands ; from which reason the fraternity considered, in comparison to them, the wisest of ordinary mankind as dolts and blockheads, and esteemed all the riches of the world, and all the accumulations of kings, as below contempt, in the face of the Rosicrucians' possible power to convert solidity itself into gold (which of course takes in everything), and to institute dealings, to their advantage, with all the worlds of the invisibles. To such men as these what could worldly riches be? On the contrary, instead of desiring worldly honours and advantages, or wishing to be even known, they ignored all human association, as sympathetic to them, and they fled from the eyes of men in their character of philosophers; but they mixed with the world familiarly in their appearance of ordinary persons, enjoying the world, and using it as a sort of play, or extravagant or brutal masquerade wherewith, to amuse. In fact, after all, and notwithstanding the wondering whispers and accounts about them, there is only the *suspicion* of the existence of these strange beings as real men; for no man in the old time, any more than in the period nearer to the present, or in the present times, can boast that he has ever been face to face, or that he has ever been in real visible converse with a Rosicrucian, or with one of these transcendently illustrious philosophers, in regard of whom it has been hazarded as a supposition that they must have been of " the council of God," in the same sense as Saint John the Divine, or Elias, or Enoch, or the Transfigured; such being the only method of explaining their supposed—their apparently preposterous pretensions. In their superlative majesty of superiority to it, and in their weariness and disgust of everything human, they even declined unbounded length of life in this world, rejecting with all possible joy the infinite

prolongation possible of life down here in this mortal
state, which (it was said of them) already lay in their
hands by the means of their famous elixir, or their magic
methods of rejuvenescence; also their command of beauty,
or of riches, and of all supernatural gifts—so surely in
their hands, but refused and ignored because of their
interpenetration of persuasion of the vanity of all life in
comparison with the never-ending, always-beginning pros-
tration, in the sense of *infinite humility*, before God, the
Almighty. In their souls they were always prostrate
before the Throne of the Almighty Creator, in whose
service alone lay the immortal rapture.

The secrets of these Sublime Brothers, the true members of the "R. C.," are no more to be divulged, than
they can be supposed accessible to even the most super-
eminent among the ordinary children of men. Indeed,
the best safeguard of the mysteries is the perfect impossibility of their ever being rendered intelligible, or,
if intelligible, of their ever being believed possible.
" Outside," and " Inside," when they contradict each
other, can assuredly never become identical, except in
supernatural possession, or in that state which men understand by that unaccounting, and unaccountable, word—
the inflow of the Holy Ghost. It is a miracle (which
must always be divine; because a miracle, otherwise than
divine, is, of course, an impossibility) wherein, in the
mind of the subject momentarily realised to it, conviction
tramples triumphantly up the impossibilities into the possible! And therein, time becomes " no time"—space
becomes " no space."

It is the hermetic theory that the shadows, lost from
this side, are not wholly gone—that the loss is not en-

tirely passed out of the magic rings, or folds, or investments of " this world's" nature, which, in reality, begins
to renew when it seems to cease; but that it is recover-
able in the magic art of the adepts, or Rosicrucians;
and that its objects can be " got back," in the exercise of
the magic, and of the adequate practice of the true
Alchemists; intent upon their object, and taken up out
of the lower world, to work in the higher.

The Rosicrucians, who explored the wonders of the
natural world, and the wonders and mysteries of the supersensual world—those supposed magicians, who forced, or
who rather *prayed,* down into the very depths of their
abasement and humility before the idea of God (and of
the rescuing, merciful, and pitying God), rising thus into
sainthood, looked upon nature with very different eyes to
ordinary philosophers.   They were enabled (spiritually)
to penetrate to the truth of the original Fall of the Angels,
and to trace the " marks" of the thunder (they needed not,
in their sense of humbleness, and " poverty of spirit," to
take warning by them) which had precipitated the overthrown rebellious Spirits from the heights, and holds, and
palaces of Heaven (under the ruling of the Arch Divinity)
to the dismal vales, and the earthquake-channelled sides of
the mountains, and the fires and darkness of the penal
Hell—their prison; the monster, mythic chains of which
are grasped in the hands of the watching Saint Michael,
the " generalissimo of the armies of Heaven;" whose
archangelic personality is figured forth, (for man's feebler
comprehension, unable to rise out of the mathematics of
the false nature, which is the parody of the real nature,)
in the blessed Saint George on earth, with his " Sanguine
Cross"—at once the talisman through heaven, and the

terror through hell, to those who can understand it. That Cross, the cognizance, and the palladium, of this land, sacred from innumerable saints, and warlike, and other holy martyrs, distinguished in the centuries of the British story—is displayed in this our country, in this England of ours! Our country will surely be obliterated, when it effaces the Cross from its emblazonments.

Nature is a term of indefinite expansion with these mysterious Rosicrucians. Their questions are very deep and incomprehensible. Of some of their ideas and theories— we speak of the Gnostics, as well as of the Rosicrucians in this place—there is only a glimpse, like a ray, to be caught now and then. The very highest capacity of mind may be tasked to arrive at the possibility of the comprehension of their religion, and to apprehend the reasonableness of some of their conclusions. Can we blame these explorers into the heights, for their jealous exclusion, when they multiply risks in the path up the mountain of light, and mark the track by innumerable purposely-placed pitfalls? Incompetent, audacious seekers earn their defeat in their attempts to follow those who are urging up. The path is most carefully, step by step behind them, obliterated by the true sons of knowledge, to those improper querists. Dare we question their wisdom, who thus deny and bar the road, and who invoke the clouds to conceal them, and the presented points of the flames as the spears of the angelic rearguard to close in and fence their march upward into the light? The story of Faust, or Doctor Faustus, and the magicians and the sages who are described in the old romances to have pined for the forbidden knowledge—these determents supply abundant warning as to this kind of dangerous ambition. This straining after the knowledge which Nature has—for the preservation of itself, be it noted—so successfully concealed and buried deep in the mysteries is, in the Miltonic sense, "dust and bitter ashes"—the "apples of Sodom," instead of the apples of the Hesperides—guarded by the Dragon; the Old Serpent, or First Rebel, be it remembered. This class of wise men, or wizards, are those who are fabled to have "sold their souls"—or the chance, or possibility, of the survival of that which the world calls their soul, out of this world—to the Fiend, the Enemy of Mankind (he is to be found in all theologies, in all ages), for wealth and honours, and long life, and a round of power and an exhaustion of sensual enjoyment, and the indulgence of the human passions for a term—to which the liberal and politic Devil was never found grudging enough to fix a limit: the most insatiate appetites were to be fully satisfied in this respect with worldly enjoyments, in all the fables bearing upon this subject:—traffickers of the sort, like Faust and his compeers, bargained for things visible in the world; exchanging white hairs and decrepitude, poverty and disdain, for wealth and unbounded power. They exchanged intoxication of delight for the horrors of despair, new life and new creation for the worn-out old ife and for the old creation, which had been exhausted, and was found only suffused with anguish and despair of all sorts. But the Rosicrucians were champions of know-ledge and of aims of a different stamp, and, despising the vain things of this life, sought for other life than this. They sought no alliance with "Traitors against Heaven." They trampled the desirable things of this lower world under foot. They had transcended out of the "dust and

ashes" of ordinary life. They were true to their names
of the "Brothers of the Red Cross." They were glorified
with a passion of grief for the accumulating sorrows, first in
the inflictions which sprang into the tempest of tears, and
at last—in the natural and supernatural rigours of the
"Garden of Agony."

The tortures and the sacrifice of Calvary—the Passion
of the Cross—were, in their glorious blessed magic and
triumph, the protest and appeal (how this should be, and
be REAL, can only be seen, of course, in the mystical
conviction of the initiates). The flowing blood streamed
from the crown, or the piercing circlet of the thorns of
Hell. The Rose is feminine. Its lustrous carmine petals
are guarded with thorns. The Rose is the most beautiful
of flowers. The Rose is the Queen of God's Garden.
It is not the Rose, alone, which is the magical idea (or
truth). But it is the "Crucified Rose," or the Martyred
Rose (by the grand mystic Apocalyptic figure), which is
the talisman, the standard, the object of adoration of all
the Sons of Wisdom, or of the true Rosicrucians.

How this latter assertion should be intelligible, and be
REAL, can only be seen, of course mystically, in the conviction of the genuine members of the R. C.

CHAPTER XIV.

THE GNOSTICS AND THEIR BELIEFS.

THE beliefs of the Gnostics are not by any means to be considered as shared by the present author, although he may seem to argue narrowly for them; or for them in certain apologetic shapes, or some free shape.

These philosophic outlines figure forth the foundation and abstract meanings, never to be taken literally, or brought too close home, of the Gnostic Left-Hand-side contemplation of Nature—a contemplation informed and illuminated, although reckoned apocryphal and heretical, and one which may, for reasons unfathomable in the philosophies, have been supernaturally suggested. Supernaturalism (that is, "Nature made by some other thing than itself") is undoubtedly true, although in the nature of things it cannot be reconciled with common sense. Common sense undoubtedly accepts, and must accept if it would be true to itself, the outside world, with which it is in contact every day; and this (truly) is the "world of things." This phrase, the "world of things," comprises all that is meant in the world, of the "things of the senses." All are "ideas," in fact—which is conception, from moment to moment, and this parade of ideas is all that is *really real.* But this cogitation within ourselves, or thought, or picture, or whatever it be—or response to shadow from outside, or effect upon the *sensorium*—will by no means prove that we are really in contact with real things. This notion has been success-

fully refuted by the profounder philosophers—even by
the profounder realists, who, like Hume and others who
believe with him, have sunk their metaphysical plummets
the deepest into reality for a foundation, and who adopt
the same obstinate processes of thinking out, or who, in
other words, split divisions between things. Thus this
question of the actual reality, or of the actual *non-reality*
of anything being existent outside and out of man, has
been left by them—wisely, in fact, because they could
not avoid the conclusion without stultifying themselves,
which in their natural, and still more in their acquired
PRIDE, they were certainly very unwilling to do. Thus
this grand question was left an open question—that is, a
question so far " open" that one can, in metaphysic
ingenuity, run any theory through it. It is built up, or
rather it is placed there by itself, as the only reliable
principle taking its spring from common sense, to be no
more contradicted than "common sense." Of a parallel
with this certainty is the spontaneous irremovable knowledge of a man who is comfortably confident that he has
not been conjured into this world by magic, but has been
born of his " mother," and begotten of his " father," to
use the rough expression, which is, after all, not true,
because the father is only the *representative* of something
else, and the generator is only a *means*, inasmuch as no
one—out of the world—can call him the cause. In fact,
there is nothing so mysterious as conception, "getting,"
gestation, and birth, and all the mysterious phenomena
which move along with each. Further on—in continued
relation to these strange Gnostic subjects—we purpose
to freely examine free subjects. And these subjects shall
be as delicately treated (which we are sure the intelligent

reader, by-and-by, will admit and confirm) as is possible, when the great aim of speaking to the point is to be attained. We have already too much verbiage and too few ideas in the world.

The treatise which we have in view is one certainly original. At first sight, the observations—or some of the observations—will seem very *free*. But we do not write for the ordinary kinds of readers. We do not write for the over-fastidious, nor for readers always prepared with their suspicions, particularly about our maintenance of what are called decencies. Our comments are not intended to be examined by the hypercritical or ultra-sensitive. For there is a false sensitiveness which is quite misplaced, and a false delicacy which is no delicacy at all, but only an ill-advised, self-distrustful, heavy, illiterate, shamefaced barbarism. Nature is nature, and nature will be nature to the end of the chapter. Try as we will to effect the elimination, that which is inseparable from nature will stick to it. And it will stick to it, sometimes, with more dangerous results after its elimination has been attempted. For in these peculiar cases it is not familiarity which breeds contempt, but familiarity which conduces to *respect*. For the means and the effect are so contradictory, and yet so grand; in the sense that whilst such and such things are ordered—such and such things are forbidden.

In all the matters treated of in this Book, in the meaning and purpose of art—such as music, particularly—the grand contention is, whether the world may be said to have SPRUNG—to apply the word thus—from feeling, or was CONSTRUCTED—so to describe the mythic making of nature—from science? In this distinction lies everything of philosophic abstraction in regard to the subjects "Power," and "Love," as originators of the scheme of things. We may put the question in other words as a theosophic speculation, whether man—and therefore art— is from the *head*, or the *heart?* We think entirely the latter, in as far as "Love" is greater than "Wisdom," and is its ruler. In this great fact of the superiority of "Love" over "Wisdom," and in the well-known truth that the one dominates the other, it appears to us, lies all the hope of the world. Through wisdom—mystically— the world would never have been. Through justice the world would never have been spared, and perpetuated. In the regard of justice, the world is naught. Mercy and love, combined and interfused, become "Immortal Pity," and therefore the means of saving it; indeed, this "Immortal Pity" alone saves the world. Therefore—in the human sense—contrition: therefore, sacrifice: therefore, submission—"like as little children:" these save it. "Verily, verily, I say unto you, unless ye become as 'little children'"—human pride and the vanity of science being trodden under foot by you—"ye shall, in no wise, see the kingdom of God." To this possible relaxing of the sternness of punishment (Justice) and the punitive (there- fore cleansing) awards of Jehovah, the Saints penetrated. This means the "Propitiation," or the sacrifice of the "Saviour," or of the sensitive, or sympathising, side of human nature, alarmed at pain, in immortal terror at the sufferings of humanity, and melting in pity at it; there- fore partaking of the pain, to invalidate the horrors of it, and resigning for the penalty, since that could be alone sufficient. In this emotion from the heart lies all religion, and all that we can know, of ourselves, of hope—of hope for humanity in this earthly state, which is clearly penal, for some original, immortal sin, of the real nature of which Man can know nothing.

In the enthusiasm of devotion, God moved thereto, and permitting it, foregoing "Wisdom" altogether, the human heart (not the HEAD, remember, the seat of the intelligence,) gives way, and pours itself instinctively out in pity—giving itself for that which it seeks to share, and, in sharing, to save. That the guilt and Fall of our First Parents, in mysterious ways, which we cannot understand, and for things and for crimes against God which we cannot understand, is true, and a real thing in the parade, and the possibilities, of that abstraction, Time, however impossible of belief in common sense, we make absolute account; in some mode, or manner, which it is impossible for the human race to understand, and which—in this earthly state—must ever transcend all possibility of the means of reaching. Christ's immortal sadness at the world (which is a ruin) may be understood in some of these mystical and remote senses. Christ's self-sacrifice in it (and for it) induced by that immortal pity—angelic, godlike, since it is spread through the ages, and as it is commensurate with the expansion of the "panoramas" of Time :—this can surely acquire justification, in faith, as a reality—if anything either in the world (or out of it) is real. Thence the "Garden of Agony." Thence the record, in the words of the Scripture—"My soul is sad, even unto tears"—(of blood !) "My soul is sad, even unto Death !"

The writings of the great mystical master, Jacob Bœhm, indicate all these phases and specialties of faith in a wonderfully subtle manner. He becomes a most engrossing writer when the attention upon him fixes intensely and his meaning has been gained ; which is no slight matter of attainment when the intricacy and the inherent obscurities of his style are considered. This illustrious man—whose writings and teachings are a puzzle to the Anglican Church, and, indeed, to all Christian Churches, whose professors are unable to rise to the heights of his spontaneous mystical sublimity, and who ignore him because they cannot understand him—was born in the year 1575, and died in 1624. His books—remarkable enough—are sought with the utmost avidity and curiosity by adepts, and the genuine editions are very difficult to be met with, particularly in English. Jacob Bœhm's Christian mysticism is, *in se* and *per se*, pre-eminently catholic, but was disallowed by the Roman Catholics, although Bœhm labours for the illustration of their chief dogmas, though not by their modes and in their own way. In all Christian respects, if (doubtless) with a Gnostic tinge, he labours grandly and zealously. Nevertheless, Jacob Bœhm, though personally a most submissive, unaggressive man—the simplest of the simple, the most innocent of the innocent—was followed up and persecuted, in spite of his appeals to the higher authorities, who always seemed to entertain some favourable doubt of whether he was right or whether he was wrong ; and he was greatly interrupted, distressed, and annoyed. Indeed, the ignorance, and consequent blind disregard, even amounting to aversion, of all the principal people, and the favourably-placed people, of the modern Protestant Church in this country, towards this strangely powerful teacher are very remarkable, and very little to their credit. It is very strange, truly, that by a religion which is disclosed as inspiring all enthusiasm, in the present exercise of the Christian religion in England, Jacob Bœhm should be so much whispered down and so greatly dreaded. But the English, especially in the modern day, are very unimpressionable, cold, and impassive.

The mystic views propounded by Jacob Bœhm in regard to the Christian scheme greatly resembled the profoundly metaphysical, far-off (stigmatised as visionary) ideas of Robert Fludd. It is impossible to suppose other than that in some form or by some means Robert Fludd was acquainted with the apocalyptic impressions and the deep religious dreaming of the great German mystic. We have innumerable proofs of this in a parallel consideration of the writings of both. Bœhm wrote inspirationally—that is, altogether from the interior vision —and he wrote from the outside impossibilities into the inside possibilities. He was an uneducated man, a poor man, a lowly man. He had no scholarship, no learning. Robert Fludd, on the contrary, was one of the most learned men of his time, with reading, scholarship, and experience widely extensive, and gathered up from all the erudite centres. There was all the difference in the world between the two great men—standing alone and unapproachable in their time in their thinking power—and yet their conclusions and notions were exactly the same, or, if they differed, differed only in degree.

A puzzle also exists in the history of Robert Fludd, the great English Rosicrucian, and the supposed founder, or discoverer, or revealer, or restorer (this latter would be the better meaning with which to invest the wonder) of Freemasonry, if we are to believe De Quincey's account of the supposed origin of Freemasonry. This puzzle arises, after all that appears as certainty, from the doubt whether there were not *two* Fludds; indeed, to come the closer in unexpected juxtaposition, even two Robert Fludds. Of this novel and singular problem in biographical identification, we offer the following solution, derived from the *Biographie Universelle*, tom. xv., p. 109, *et supra*.

"*Quelques bibliographes ont confondu Robert Flood* (of Bersted, in Kent, in the Elizabethan time), *avec un autre Robert, dominicain Anglais, né à York, et qui florissait dans le* 14e *siècle. Ce religieux avait fait aussi des recherches et laissé des écrits, sur les Mystères de la Nature, ce qui l'avait fait surnommer '*Perscrutator*' (le Chercheur). Jean Pits et Jacques Echard, d'après Jean Leland, lui attribuent :* De impressionibus aeris; de mirabilibus elementorum ; de magia ceremoniali ; de mysteriis secretorum ; et correctorium alchymiæ." All these studies and subjects closely correspond, certainly, with those on account of which the real and undoubted Robert Fludd, or Flood, became justly famous. It is impossible to tell now who this first Robert Flood was, or whether he was, or was not, an ancestor of the second.

The sect called the Gnostics* included a large number

---

* *The Gnostics : Classic and Mediæval*, by the Rev. C. W. King. London : 1865.

This work is a mere cold transcript of the historical side of the characteristics of the various orders of the famous and much-reprobated Gnostics. It is necessarily poor and insufficient in attempting to treat, *with no knowledge*, of the important mystic peculiarities which distinguish these fanciful philosophers. The accounts of the Gnostics by this author, who wholly fails to grasp their meaning, are, of course, prejudiced, since he deals with the subject simply from the orthodox of professing Christians, and their doctrines were maintained by a succession of professors—called by them apostles—who spread them so zealously abroad in different parts of the Gentile world that in many places they were considered as the only people belonging to the religion of the Cross, and their conduct and beliefs the only rule by which its morality could be estimated. The Gnostics have left no account of themselves. They are known to have written some books, but the stream of time has brought down none to the present day. Their opinions, therefore, would have perished, perhaps, with themselves, many centuries ago, were they not preserved and embodied in the works of contemporary Christian writers. Irenæus has detailed their doctrines, and Epiphanius, who himself had been a Gnostic, relates their rites and practices. Besides these, several other fathers of the Church give an account of the lives and doctrines of the sect, with members of which they were personally acquainted. Some modern writers have taken up the cause of the Gnostics, and in various manners, and as cautiously as they could, have declared that they have been greatly misrepresented, and that many among those who claimed to be orthodox have in some instances, and

and academic standpoint. In a word, the Rev. C. W. King handles his great subject like most men of the Church when they write upon these matters—in a perfunctory, self-assured spirit. He criticises like a mere collector and comparer of medals, coins, gems, and so forth—a barren archæologist. The book, however, is furnished with engravings of some of the best known talismans and gems of the Gnostics, more or less authentic and curious; but these illustrations, instead of being well executed, are very rough and inelegant—a fatal fault to the force of these things. By such inconclusive means there was exhibited no knowledge of what is meant by these, in reality, wondrous tokens—the only revelation of the secret ideas of these strangely profound thinkers.

because of prejudice and malevolence—instigated by fear
of the powers of thought of the Gnostics—vilified them,
and traduced their principles and designs, and that in
other and more mischievous instances, they have failed
utterly to understand them or to grasp their courage of
aim and their directness of clear sight and reasoning.
That the Gnostics were very ambitious thinkers, and
philosophers of a profound and an extended range of
investigation, there can be no doubt. In fact, some of
their ideas alarmed the general mind, as laying the
axe to the root of all authentic consciousness and responsibility. They were accused of entertaining dogmas
which could not be worked with success in a world which
was clearly never intended for aberration from standards,
nor for the speculations which must ruinously result from
the reveries of these strange men.

Some writers of the modern time, who bear the pious
fathers of the Church no goodwill, seek every occasion
to throw discredit upon the testimony of the ecclesiastical
commentators upon the doctrines of the Gnostics, as they
stand expressed or implied, avowed or suspected. Accordingly these bolder writers represent the Gnostics, not
as they are depicted by those who stand forward as
having seen or known them, but as men of high intellectual attainments, sublime in their views, rational in
their opinions, and pure in their conversation. These
dissentients to the accepted Christian ideas accuse the
orthodox of arguing for a narrow Christian philosophy,
and of assuming too low grounds—nay, of forming a total
misconception of the true nature and veritable scope
of the great Christian idea. They accuse the Christians,
pure and simple, of a low-minded pureness, and truly of

a simplicity, not simple in the large sense, but simple in the small sense. They say that the minds of these people are not lofty enough—they assert that ordinary Christians are incapable of viewing the true Christian ideas as abstractions, or of rising into real spirituality or transcendentalism. They maintain that ordinary theologians— in fact, that all who entertain a different opinion to those opinions to which they themselves profess to have attained —are full of conclusions derived from prejudice and incredulity, similar to the Scriptural "hardness of heart" which carries with it a parallel "hardness of the understanding," imputed to the oblivious and reluctant Hebrews —impatient, as not understanding what they were told. The famous Gnostic gems, the wonder and the puzzle of all commentators upon the mysteries of the Gnostics, are the only monuments the Gnostics themselves have transmitted of their daring imaginations and principles suspected in some quarters as licentious.

Some of the finest and grandest (not fine or grand in the sense of finish or execution, but in the ideas which they suggest—although only to the capable, which necessitates large knowledge—and of the sublime mysteries of which they speak, and to which they are whispered to refer) are given, in reproduction, in this present work, and have been selected with the greatest care and with cautious judgment. These are confidently submitted to the observation of those persons elevated in mind and of a philosophical and curious turn. But it must not be supposed that the execution of these Gnostic gems, or coins, or objects is necessarily beautiful or excellent. In fact, in the majority of instances, it is quite the reverse. Some even, at first consideration of them,

seem barbarous and unintelligible, being bewildering
and not answering to any apparently reasonable idea.
This may convince as all the more natural considering
that the very purpose of these gems, or tokens, or marks,
or coins is a matter of doubt and debate, and that they
are most known as talismans and amulets, of course
carrying the idea of charms and spells, and bringing in
the impressions of magic and magic speculations and
supernatural powers, whether derived from holy or
unholy sources, with them, and obtruding all this into
the ordinary world of man, disturbing it with " thoughts
beyond the reaches of his soul."

Thus the Gnostics have been always regarded as
uncomfortable philosophers, truly, as their name implies,
" knowing," and perhaps " knowing too much," bringing
a weight of mystery with them, and impressing us as
those strange and unaccountable movers through the
world, regarding whom history speaks with subdued
breath and romance tells exciting tales—persons in regard
of whom one walks out of the way, whose time of
appearance is twilight, whose advent is pre-denoted by
murmurs of thunder, whose movements are wayward,
whose comings and goings are perplexing, whose address
is fantastic and yet fearful, and who must be regarded
with distrust, if not with apprehension and absolute
suspicion. Such were the Gnostics—at all events, in the
usual orthodox Christian view. Such were also those
renowned, discredited characters, the Rosicrucians, in
the popular idea. Thus it must always be with remarkable characters and great men.

These philosophers assumed the appellation of Gnostics
in the self-sufficient and enthusiastic belief that they

enjoyed a more intimate acquaintance with the Divine
nature and a profounder insight into religious mysteries
than was vouchsafed to the rest of the Christian world.
They were, almost without exception, of the Gentile
race, and their principal founders seem to have been
natives of Syria and Egypt. The paths of speculation
being various and infinite, the Gnostics were imperceptibly
divided into more than fifty particular sects, of which the
most celebrated appear to have been the Basilideans, the
Valentinians, and the Marcionites. They first became
conspicuous in the second century, after the death of the
apostles, and under the reign of the Emperor Hadrian;
they flourished during the third century, and were superseded, for the most part, in their importance in the
fourth or fifth. The Oriental philosophy was the
principal fountain from which they drew their ideas.
The rational soul, or conscious entity, according to that
refining philosophy, was imprisoned in corrupt matter
contrary to the will of the Supreme Being, and the world
was subject to the dominion of a number of evil genii, or
malignant spirits. To liberate the soul from her thral-
dom and emancipate the human race from the tyranny of
these demons, the Eastern sages expected the coming
of an extraordinary messenger from the Most High.
The followers of the Gnostic religion reduced the facts
and doctrines of the Gospel into conformity with their
Oriental tenets. Their notions concerning Jesus Christ
were as follows:—They considered Him as the Son of
God, but they denied both His deity and His humanity,
the former because they identified Him with the visionary
deliverer of their Eastern superstition, the latter because
they held everything corporeal to be intrinsically and

essentially evil. It was inconsistent with their ideas of
the human body to believe that so impure a tabernacle
was prepared for a good being, who came to destroy the
empire of wicked spirits and restore the souls of men into
a state of union with the great source from which they
emanated. It was a farther result of their tenets with
regard to matter that they rejected the doctrine of the
resurrection, or the reunion of soul and body after death.
The same deterrent and suspicious opinions led also
to other irregular physiological conclusions. Some of
the professors of the Gnostic form of belief were such
particular and impossible purists that they looked with
displeasure at the incitements of the flesh which
led to propagation; and they failed to see the truth in
Nature that the whole of the mechanical perfections of
man's body tend up to the securing of the completest
success in this matter of the winning representatives, as
also that woman's form is expressly built up, converging
at the waist evidently for the purpose of showing to what
purpose the woman was constructed, the body of the
woman incontestably foreshadowing, in its slopes upwards
and downwards to the centre, the direct object to fortify,
to sustain, and to maintain for the bearing and the bringing forth of progeny. Wherefore comes all this pre-
vision and all this mechanical exactness, combined with
all-powerful allurements, if not for the one overriding and
principal object—that of safeguard and perpetuation of
the race? Nature presents this as the grand object, and,
as it would seem, almost as the *only* object of life, not the
individual being, the object of all begetting or reproduction, but the simple fact of securing continuity; even
as a sort of beautiful and grand punishment of "waste:"

this world being a sort of method of being, of purgatory
or punishment for some nameless sins in some other place
or state, the whole history and account of which, and the
reasons for which, have been purposely hidden away from
man's knowledge, or have been lost. The reader will
perceive that we are arguing that this world is not the
proper world of man, and that, according to the ideas of
the Buddhists, man is not in a proper world at all, but
that he is the victim of the deceitful investments, visions
in circles on circles, but yet real and material, as he takes
them to be; man being "asleep," as it were, "for
thousands of years," and being, in his historical periods
and in his processes of sensation, "not in reality at all,"
but only passing on unconsciously as the sport of the
delusions of the inveterate "Maya." This was a strange,
shadowy belief, but it was the real philosophy and the
only one relied upon by the genuine Gnostics, and also
closely assimilating to the profound metaphysical deductions of the Buddhists, whose philosophy was precursory
to that of the Platonists, everything originally, not only
the religions, but the nations, coming from the East, and
working gradually westwards, as if obeying a grand law
of Nature, which should pass all *phenomena* in the way of
the rolling of the world. The world was peopled westward. All civilisation has proceeded and intensified, in
the course of the generations, westward; and progress has
made its march with the sun. Thus we are witnessing,
perhaps, "the last rally" (so to use the word) of the
over-elaborated and extravagant and debased hyper-
civilisation of this "Dispensation," culminating oppres-
sively, even offensively, in the uprising multitudinous
centres of the "Far West" of the prodigious continents

of the two Americas, stretching nearly from pole to pole on the West board, and facing again that (metaphorically speaking) worm-eaten hive of old formal grandeurs and of the old scientific elaborations of ancientest and most fixed and fossilised civilisation—China, with its millions (with a far-off meaning) of curious microscopical creatures, a race, or races, which, in certain quaint senses, can hardly be pronounced human; at least as we Westerns understand humanity; the ingenuities of these marvellous Chinese being of that peculiar character that they seem short, even from their fixedness and finish, of perfection, and in their inexpansiveness and unimpulsiveness, of human. And yet—actually to say and to add to the wonder—in this monumental Cathay, which seems, from its foundation, to have worked through the *eras* in a sort of a dream as of a "tutelary toyshop," socially and historically, or, as in the rigidities of a mythologised "Noah's Ark," with all its princes and patriarchs, and all its animals and habitudes, really, in this old China, wherein—without meaning it as a joke—the quaint people seem, in the eternal iteration of their forms and manners and customs, to work back-wards, and not to beget sons as Nature seems to expect of the generations, but actually to give again the birth into the world of their grandfathers, acting under the dictates of a blind perverse mechanism—here, at the last margin of the world eastward, we encounter the most incontrovertible traces of the universal Phallicism, or worship and deification of the human apotheosised, sexual, magical "means" and "instruments" (made images and symbols of the gods). These we recognise in felicitous disguises, not only in the temples and at every corner of the streets of every Chinese city and town, but magnificently and beautifully in the many-storied pagodas, dotted all over with tinkling bells; in the carvings and eaves and cornices, in the silks and strings, in the *umbos* and umbrellas, in all the embellishments throughout China, outdoors and indoors, inundated all over with every form of mythological zoology,—namely, renderings of dragon-bird, dragon-beast, or dragon-fish.

China seems to be populated and to be instinct, in the lively recollections of those happy travellers who have visited it, with eternal images lustrous in the gold of the grand golden Sun, or Dragon of Yellow Fire, recalling the one superb idolatry which may be specified as that of "*Bells* and the Dragon." The Chinese pagodas are, in truth, no other than veritable Tors or Phalli, of the same character as those found all over the earth. All these speak the same story and convey the same meaning as the Irish Round Towers, as all the towers of India, as all the minarets of the Mahometans, as all the obelisks in Egypt and elsewhere, as the Great Pyramid—nay, all pyramids and pyramidical structures, as the rough single stones and corneds and cromlechs, and stone pillars and stone crosses, as the circles of stones, and groups of memorial stones, and votive stones, as the menhirs of Brittany, as the carns or cairns—as Carnac in the West of France, as Stonehenge and Abury, or Avebury, in England; as the universal "Tors" and architectural rounds; nay, to sum up the whole parade of exemplars from the original "Babel," to the last church tower or spire raised yesterday in any part of the world, or from the "pillow-stone"—sacred and blessed—which the patriarch Jacob took and set on end as his "pillar"-stone, or motive-mark, or altar of acknowledgment to

Jehovah, when he "awoke from out of his dream," and acknowledged with awe that "God had been there," to the Western Steeples, even to the familiar western steeples of Saint Paul's Cathedral in our own over-powering wilderness or world of a capital, this mighty metropolis, London.

As matter was evil in its nature, so, according to the Gnostics, it was evil in its source. The material world, in their system, was the creation of those bad genii who governed it; and the direct consequence of this notion was that they denied the divine authority of the Old Testament, whose account of the beginning of things was so totally repugnant to their peculiar theories. They even went so far as to view Moses, and the religion he taught, with abhorrence. In the God of the Jews they could discover none of the features of the wise and omni-potent Father of the Universe; and, accordingly, they degraded Him to a lower order of existence, sometimes even so low as the evil principle itself.

The moral doctrines of the Gnostics were of two kinds, and those diametrically opposite to each other. The lives of those of one class were austere and abstinent; they mortified and attenuated the body, in order to purify and elevate the mind. The other class maintained that there was no moral difference between human actions. And, in conformity with this principle, they gave free course to their passions, and made religion itself minister to their sensual gratifications. These doctrines, apparently so opposite, had their origin in the same principle, operating on different characters and temperaments. The body being universally accounted the source and seat of evil, men of morose and stern dispositions sought to reduce and combat it, as the natural enemy of the soul; while, on the other hand, persons of dissolute propensities were easily brought to believe that the deeds of the outward man had no relation whatever to the state of the inward, and that, consequently, the idea of moral restraint upon the former was absurd.

It may be doubtful whether the Gnostics of the rigid or those of the sensual school did most to prejudice the cause of Christianity in the eyes of the heathen world. The religion of the gospel is as far from being a code of austere discipline and rigid observances as it is from sanctioning the vices and passions of our corrupt nature.

We have said that the Gnostics first acquired celebrity in the second century; their first appearance, however, in ecclesiastical history belongs to an earlier date, and has been traced satisfactorily even so far back as the apostolic times. At the period when the gospel was first promulgated, the practice of magic, and the belief in the powers of certain men in this respect, was general in every part of the civilised world; and there cannot be a doubt that the more important nations had attained to the highest possible point of perfection, and of civilisation, in all the arts of living. The popular creed, and the highly-wrought imagination of the educated, the skilful, and the luxurious— nay, the notions of the speculators and the philosophers, in the necessities of things, and in the visible and believed abounding richness of nature—peopled all the regions conceivable, real and unreal, "earth, air, flood, and fire," with certain influences and powers which could be appealed to, and managed and swayed, for good or for evil, by the proficient in the use of spells and charms, mystical sounds and emblems.

The Egyptians were proverbial for cherishing these wild impressions of the possibilities of penetrating to and of holding commerce with the unknown, and of operating upon the true faculties of spirits and entities—more or less communicative, or disposed, or not indisposed, to be communicative, and even to benefit by traffic with men and women. These degrees and orders of spirits were farther imagined to partake in the gift and endowment, or in the depravation and punishment by the Supreme Power—working through all matter by means of its representatives and ministers. These spirits were also supposed to be capable of human characteristics. The life of all nature was imagined to be conscious and penetrative. The senses were only the means of analysis of a general grand magic intelligence—an intelligence which, diffused through nature, was infiltrated through universal being, and operated in man in various influenced modes, in regard of which he was totally unaware of the spring or object; nor could he guess whither he was drifting in the directions, and in the sinuosities of astrology—where the smallest should introduce to the greatest, and the greatest should bring about, and terminate and act in the smallest:—all obeying a certain extended supernatural scheme, of which man could surmise neither the particular drift nor the general purpose. Nor was man equal, in his limited faculties, to guessing the meanings of nature—this being in the hands—not even of the inferior, but only of the high-placed gods, in the ascending chain of degrees even up to the Highest.

The Egyptians were proverbial for entertaining the most singular prepossessions in regard to being, fate, necessity, charms, science, and magic—this last, sinister

and malevolent as exercised by the envious and malicious
preternatural powers; as also good, rescuing, and benevolent, when interposed, as a means of extrication, by the
agents, or angels, of the great good genius, or merciful
master of universal nature.   We find, in the Acts of the
Apostles, that the study of "curious arts" was common
amongst the inhabitants of the most polished city of the
East.   It is not surprising, therefore, that many of the
first converts to the Cross should have corrupted the
purity of the new creed with a profane mixture of their
ancient habits and ideas.   Simon Magus is by many
writers considered as the father of all the Gnostic heresies.
He had been (or is assumed to have been) a wizard by
profession; and so persuaded were the people that he
was some extraordinary person that they affirmed him to
be " the great power of God" (Acts viii. 9, 10).   It is
asserted that he was converted by Philip's preaching, and
that he believed and was baptised.   However this may
be, it is said of him that he relapsed soon after into his
old ways, and we find that he is reported to have proffered
money to Peter and John, to be endued, like them, with
the power of working miracles.   The terrible rebuke
which this impious proposal met with brought him, for a
season, to a penitent frame of mind.   Here, however,
the apostolic narrative leaves him; and, to complete his
history, we must refer to other sources of information.
We learn from Origen that he was at Rome during the
persecutions under Nero; that he taught his followers
that they might conform to the rites of Paganism without
sin; and that, by this latitudinarian doctrine, he saved
them from the cruelties perpetrated on their more con-
scientious brethren.   (*Origen adv. Celsum*, lib. vi.)   All

that we know further of this personage favours the opinion
of Mosheim, that he is rather to be placed amongst the
open enemies of Christianity than in the number of those
who corrupted and impaired it. (Mosheim, *Eccles. Hist.*,
vol. i., p. 140.) In fact, he not only deserted the
Christian religion (if, by the way, he ever joined it), but
openly opposed it; nay, he went so far as to announce
himself as the Saviour of the world. Nor was this
enough. He is said to have asserted that he united in his
own nature all the persons of the Trinity; in Samaria,
his native country, he was the Father; in Judæa, the Son;
amongst the Gentiles, the Holy Spirit. (*Irenæus*, lib. i.,
c. 20. *Epiphanius*, 21.) All the enormities of this supposed magician need not be related; one, however, is too
singular to be omitted:—he carried about with him a
woman named "Helena," and announced her as the identical person whose fatal beauty had occasioned the Trojan
war. She had passed through a hundred transmigrations
into her present form; she was the first conception, he
said, of his own eternal mind (in a pre-state, that he
recognised, of his own sentience); by her he had begotten
angels and archangels; and by these had the world been
created. The disciples of Magus represented him in the
form of Jupiter, and his female associate under that of
Minerva (or "holy power," producing, in magic, "holy
wisdom," and both eventuating in visible forms, or forms
of flesh). Some ideas of this sort are undoubtedly indicated in the first of those Gnostic amulets which afterwards became so varied and so mysterious. One of these
Dr. Walsh thinks is likely to have been fabricated by the
immediate followers of Simon Magus. The stone is
chalcedony, and the sculpture rude. Jupiter is repre-

sented in armour, an image of victory in his hand, and
the eagle and thunderbolt at his feet. On the reverse is
an inscription which has not been explained. However,
the ideas of all the Gnostics were suffused deeply and
inextricably with Phallicism, and with the profundities and
mysteries of Phallicism—which, in fact, is the golden key
to unlock all the treasuries of the sacred controversialists,
and the theologians and theosophists, and interpenetrates
all the reveries of the philosophers of the deeply-thinking
Gnostic order:—men who really did construct Christianity
from the grand point of view. For the true Gnostics
were philosophers who borrowed out of the " extended
spaces" (to use a figure) of " sublimity," and conjured
the fires of the abstruser magic into the brightest lights,
to illuminate the " structures" disclosed to the " dreams"
of man from amidst them; to reveal to the world (albeit
only for moments), in inspired recognition, the abode of
the greater Divinities,* who vouchsafed the " Sensible
Existence." This " Sensible Existence" is to be accepted
and interpreted in the Buddhistic sense:—Buddhism
being the first, and the foundation of all the theologies,
taking its stand (for earth, and for earthly comprehension)
on Phallicism—celestial in the first instance, terrestrial
eventually; and witnessed to in the architectural monuments of the whole world, in all ages, and amidst all peoples.
This is seen in all the varieties of steeple, and tower
and turret; all the forms of pyramid and obelisk; all the
secret symbols ventured by the sage builders; all the

---

* We must eliminate all ideas of indecency in regard to the Phallic
convictions and the Phallic worship before we become qualified to take
in, or even realise, the possibility of these ideas, which are undoubtedly
strange and difficult of belief.

"double-meaning" tokens and *insignia* hazarded in coins, talismans, and medals. All are talismans, recognised and "hailed" by the "knowing ones," which pass, every day, as through the world unseen, and as if borne in the hands of an invisible army.

The singular arrangement of the letters in the Gnostic amulet or talisman, to which we have before made reference, is supposed to be expressive of the coil of a serpent, that favourite Gnostic emblem, which is found in various forms and combinations upon most of their talismanic remains, and of which instances continually occur.

Menander, who appeared in the reign of Vespasian, had many disciples at Antioch. It appears, from the testimonies of Irenæus, Tertullian, and Justin Martyr, that he pretended to be one of the *æons*, or benevolent principles, sent from the *pleroma*, or heavenly habitation, to succour the souls that lay in bondage, and maintain them against the fraud and force of the *demons* who swayed the earth. As, therefore, he did not so much corrupt the religion which Christ taught, as set himself up in his place as a Redeemer sent from God, we must acquiesce in the opinion of Mosheim, that Menander, no more than Simon, is properly to be ranked among the Gnostics of the first century.

The claim, however, of the Nicolaitans to that appellation is undisputed. These sectaries, who defiled the church at Pergamos, and whom Christ, by the mouth of his apostle, mentions with reprobation, are supposed to have derived their origin from Nicholas, one of the seven deacons, a proselyte of Antioch. The gross licentiousness of their practice we have upon the authority of the divine Saviour (*Revelation* ii. 6, 14, 15); their questionable opinions are testified by many of the fathers, Irenæus, Tertullian, Clement, and others, who tell us that their belief embraced the doctrine of the good and evil principles—the *æons*, the origin of the world from the hands of inferior spirits, and generally all the ideas which have been mentioned as the prevailing tenets of the Gnostics. Their immorality is described to have been as revolting as their opinions were fantastical. They held sensual pleasure to be the true blessedness of man, and the great end for which he was created. The Nicolaitans soon lost the name of their founder, and branched out into a variety of new sects, all equally distinguished for extravagant principles and dissolute behaviour. It has been stated that the Gnostics were generally Gentiles. Cerinthus is an exception to this remark. He was by birth a Jew; and the religious scheme which he formed and promulgated was an amalgamation or combination of Christianity, Judaism, and the Oriental superstitions already described. The substance of this wild creed is thus given by Mosheim:—" He taught that the Creator of this world, whom he considered also as the sovereign of the Jewish people, was a Being endowed with the greatest virtues, and derived his birth from the Supreme God; that this Being fell, by degrees, from his native virtue and primitive dignity; that the Supreme God, in consequence of this, determined to destroy his empire, and sent upon earth, for this purpose, one of the ever-happy and glorious *æons*, whose name was CHRIST; that this CHRIST chose for his habitation the person of JESUS, a man of the most illustrious sanctity and justice, the son of Joseph and Mary; and, descending in the form of a dove, entered into him while he was receiving the baptism

of John in the waters of Jordan; that Jesus, after his
union with Christ, opposed himself with vigour to the
God of the Jews, and was, by his instigation, seized and
crucified by the Hebrew chiefs; that, when Jesus was
taken captive, Christ ascended up on high, so that the
man Jesus alone was subjected to the pains of an igno-
minious death." Cerinthus, farther, held the doctrine of
the millennium : Christ, he maintained, would one day
return upon earth, renew his former union with the man
Jesus, and reign with his people for a thousand years.
Such were the principal varieties of Gnosticism as it manifested itself in the first century.

Basilides, Carpocrates, and Valentine or Valentinian,
are the most eminent names among the Egyptian Gnostics.
Basilides was a native of Alexandria, and flourished about
the year 125 of the Christian era. In the singularity
and boldness of his doctrines he surpassed all his pre-
decessors. In his theological system there was one
Supreme God, from whose substance had issued seven
glorious existences, or æons. Two of these æons, Power
and Wisdom, engendered the heavenly hierarchy, or the
angels of the first order. From these was produced a
new angelic generation, of a nature somewhat less exalted.
This, in its turn, produced another, still lower in degree;
and every successive order created for itself a new heaven,
until the number of celestial descents, and of their respective heavens, amounted to three hundred and sixty-five.
Over all these presided the Supreme God, whom Basilides
hence called ABRAXAS, the letters of that word, according
to the Greek method of numeration, representing the
number 365. No term occurs more frequently than this
upon the Gnostic gems.

We proceed to the account given by Basilides of the creation of the world. The lowest order of angels had built their heaven upon the confines of matter, or rather they had constructed it out of " matter," or " darkness," as the Rosicrucian theosophy framed the idea ; "darkness," or "matter," being the lees, siftings, or *residuum*, the "accursed subsidence" of the materials, out of which alone, according to the Rosicrucians, could be obtained the " means" to construct the world, or " conjure up"— for the whole of it is magic—" nature." The whole of the creation—according to the cabalistic speculators—was the result of the gigantic " Rebellion in Heaven," and was brought about by, and incident to, the conquest of the ambitious but overthrown adverse hierarchy, thus stripped of their first celestial glory of " light," as the sons of God; which investing glory of " light" was then changed into the redness of the fierce " fires" of the penal Hell—or place of dole and doom. These ideas—be it noted—are to be found, in some form or other, more or less refined—and therefore true—in every religion which was ever instituted under Heaven ; therefore there can be no question with regard to their solidity, if real truth be a possibility at all :—which is, after all, doubtful— for the components of truth can be taken to pieces, and scattered out of the only receptacle in which truth can find hold, or refuge—namely, in the human reason :—since, out of the human reason, there is not, there never was, nor can there ever be anything. For, take the reason, or rather the sense of " self" of the " Man" away, and the whole world disappears ! The Gnostics were fully sensible of all this. They were the closest of the philosophers, who had hunted Nature out of all her secret places and resorts. They had come suddenly on Nature—surprising her as the mythological Actæon broke unpreparedly upon the sight of the matchless, awful splendour of beauty of the naked Diana. He had his reward in being marked, or "attired," as the heralds call it, with the "horns;" and the Gnostics, in a certain sense, and by a rough sort of figure, for coming upon Nature and detecting her—"behind the scenes"—contriving her tricks, have been branded and pointed at, through the Christian generations, as the most awful of heretics, and the most flagitious of men—even magicians and reprobates, owning no allegiance, nor even admitting either God or devil. That this is erroneous we all may be assured. If anything, the error lay the other way; for the Gnostics peopled all space with spirits, and referred everything to enchantments, and to the wielders and workers of the enchantments—the Enchanters.

But to return to the ideas of the Gnostics concerning the creation. They asserted—mystically, of course—that it was the lower order of angels who built their heaven upon the confines of matter, and that they soon conceived the design of moulding it into a habitable globe, and creating a race of beings to people it. Animal life was all they had to communicate to their creatures; but God, approving their plan, added a reasonable soul; and mankind, thus created, became the absolute property of the spirits whose pleasure had first called it into existence. The links which connected this extremely bold scheme with the Christian dispensation were fashioned with the same apparently profane hardihood of invention. The angelic architects of the visible world became corrupted by their familiarity with matter; they had been too conversant with clay—the vapours of the earth went up and tarnished their bright essences; hence, they fell from their heavenly character, and, waxing jealous of the Supreme Being, sought to diminish his glory and advance their own. The true knowledge of his divine nature, which he had stamped upon the human mind, they sought to obliterate. Their hands were, also, against each other; and they shook the nations with their contests for dominion. The fiercest and proudest of these degenerate spirits was the God of the Jewish people. It was principally to quell his turbulence, and overthrow his empire, that the Supreme (in compassion for mankind, which groaned under his sceptre) sent forth his Son, the chief of the *æons*, who incorporated himself with the man Jesus to execute his great commission. The demon deity prepared for his defence— his ministers went forth—the man Jesus fell into their hands and was put to death; but against Christ all their malice and fury spent themselves in vain. According to Irenæus, Basilides denied the reality of Christ's body, and held that Simon, of Cyrene, suffered in his stead. Mosheim is of opinion that some of his disciples, not himself, taught this doctrine. Basilides did not invent, but adopted, the word ABRAXAS, which represented the chief deity of the Gnostics; whose personality, and his attributes, are to be found indicated mystically upon every Gnostic gem. This mythic name—ABRAXAS—represented the number of days in the solar revolution; it stood, in the old symbolical language of Egypt, for the sun itself, the lord and governor of the heavens. From thence the Gnostics of that country transferred it to the God of their demi-pagan, demi-Christian, system.

The above account affords a comprehensive view of the

Christianity of Basilides. He taught, moreover, the Pythagorean doctrine of the transmigration of the soul, which he limited, however, to the spirits of wicked men; and he imitated the Samian sage in another particular also, for he prescribed taciturnity to his followers.* Hence the figure of Silence is found upon many of the Gnostic gems. A facsimile is given of one of these talismans, imposing silence, in the collection of Lord Strangford. Dr. Walsh notices it in his essay on the Gnostics. On one face of this coin is a female with a finger upon her lips; on the other appears the Egyptian deity, Anubis, with the head of a dog. The characters upon both faces are equally obscure.

Basilides and his followers entertained the most extravagant opinion of their superiority to all other Christian sects in divine knowledge. They only were *men*, and to hold communion with the rest of the world was to " cast their pearls before *swine*." According to Origen and Ambrosius, Basilides composed a gospel to give greater weight and currency to his opinions. Gibbon informs us that the Gnostics of his school declined the palm of martyrdom. " Their reasons," he adds, " were singular and abstruse." With respect to the morality of this great heretic, or rather of his doctrines, there exists considerable difference of opinion amongst the learned. The irregular lives of many of his disciples are, however, beyond dispute. His son, Isodorus, composed a " Treatise upon Morals," which is spoken of by the fathers as " cloaca omnium impuritatum"—a sink of all uncleanness.

Carpocrates, also of Alexandria, may be judged of by the language of Baronius, who says that he shrinks from

* Eusebius.

the recital of his tenets and practices as too shocking for Christian ears, "*ob turpitudinem portentosam nimium et horribilem*"—on account of their monstrous and revolting abominations. He differed from the sect of Basilides only in the bolder blasphemies of his creed and the far more enormous excesses of his practice. He and his disciples believed themselves to resemble Christ in all things, except that they were infinitely more powerful, for the demons were subject to their enchantments and bound to serve them. His *moral* tenets not only permitted sensuality and crime, but recommended and inculcated them. Eternal salvation, he maintained, was only within the reach of those who had daringly filled up the measure of iniquity. Our lusts and appetites were implanted by God himself, and had, therefore, nothing criminal in them. The only sin was in opposing their impulses; those who did so would be punished by the passage of their souls into other bodies; those who obeyed their desires and passions would ascend above the angels to the bosom of God the Father. In support of these atrocious dogmas he was not backward to cite Scripture. The text, "Agree with thine adversary quickly, whilst thou art in the way with him, lest he deliver thee to the judge," he interpreted as an injunction to yield to every carnal inclination. The practice of Carpocrates and his sect was not behind their doctrine. "Shall I blush only to tell what they do not blush to do?" is the indignant expression of Epiphanius while he recites their almost incredible excesses. Their Pascal feast, the least foul and disgusting of their religious rites, is described as a banquet of obscenity and horror.

The *Ophites*, or *Serpentinians*, present a remarkable variety of the Egyptian Gnostics. They followed, in

general, the system of Valentine, but they added the
monstrous tenet that the serpent (from which they took
their name) was either Christ Himself or Wisdom disguised in the form of the serpent. At first view it is
difficult to conceive by what perversion of ideas so out-
rageous a doctrine could have been invented or received.
A little reflection, however, shows that it flowed easily
from that part of the system which separated the Supreme
Being from the creator of the world, and represented the
latter as in rebellion against the former. The serpent,
therefore, in tempting the mother of mankind, could not
but be an object of veneration, for by so doing he was
shaking to its basis the kingdom of the Demiurge. We
learn from Augustine and others that the Ophites were
not content with the abstract worship of their grovelling
divinity. The serpent, we have already mentioned, was
a favourite emblem of the Gnostics; whether Greek or
Roman, African or Asiatic, they were equally disposed to
adopt the figure of that mysterious creature and to render
it as a princely potency, in the contemplative and visionary
way, in their mystic schemes, all the nations of antiquity
regarding it with similar feelings of awe and veneration.
Accordingly no device is more common upon the Gnostic
amulets.

Mosheim also mentions a Gnostic sect which held that
the *plenitude* of divine truth resided in the Greek alphabet, and that on this account Jesus Christ was designated
the Alpha and Omega.

Saturninus, Cerdo, and Marcion were the chief apostles
of the Asiatic Gnosticism, to which we proceed now to
direct the reader's attention. Saturninus was contemporary with St. Ignatius, and taught with great success at

Antioch. He held the doctrine of two eternal principles, the one good, the other evil. The latter was identical with matter, and called the material principle, or that of darkness. Seven angels, who presided over the seven planets, were the architects of the world. When the work of creation was completed, the good principle smiled upon it and blessed it, and, as the first token of his favour, he gave a reasonable soul to the inhabitants of the new earth. He then parted it equally among the seven creating angels, whose government was the natural construction of the astrological system, by the means of the harmonious going of which, or the music of the spheres, according to the teaching of Pythagoras, the world was reduced, in the hands of the gods, into the beautiful order in which it has gone on growing and invigorating. Among the seven creating angels was one who became the most powerful of all, and who was the God of the Hebrew people. This was the " Saturn" of the mythologists, and he was venerated among the Jews by the dedication to him of the seventh day, or the Sabbath—the " Saturday," the "Saturn's Day" amongst the Scandinavians. According to these dark myths the Sovereign Disposer of All Things, or the "Supreme," retained in His own hands the lordship, or the superiority of the "King of Kings," over all. Had it depended upon the good principle alone, all mankind would have been wise and just, or this state of the world, or this world altogether, *would have been impossible*, as must, in the philosophic sense, be readily seen. The "Adversary,"however—or, in fact, "DIFFERENCE"— " Two" instead of " One"—happened to assert his power. The world, or " The Word," was " made flesh," and had sunk under the law which had necessitated the fall, or the depravation, or the necessity of "the generations." This was the origin of the moral difference which we see amongst men. Ages rolled on, and in the course of the immortal, theosophic, angelic history the angelic governors of the world at length fell from their allegiance and suffered the affairs of the earth to run into disorder. Then the Good Principle sent a Restorer, whose name was Christ, and who came arrayed in the *semblance* of a human body, to destroy the empire of the Principle of Evil, and to point out to virtuous souls the way by which they must return to whence they came. Saturninus was not a sensual Gnostic. His extraordinary ideas and his resolution chose the opposite extreme of continual penance and mortification. This was the *way*, he asserted, pointed out by Christ himself. The soul could return to God by no other process save abstinence from wine, meat, wedlock—"in short, everything," says Mosheim, "that tends to sensual gratification or even bodily refreshment." Rigid as the fanaticism of this man was, he gained many proselytes; but it is manifest how the truth of Christianity must have suffered from the ridicule and odium which fell upon those whose practice was not less abhorrent to the precepts of the Gospel than inconsistent with reason and injurious to society.

Marcion held the doctrine of the two eternal principles of good and evil, but he interpolated a deity of a *mixed nature*, who was the God of the Jews and the creator of the world. This intermediate being was at perpetual feud with the evil principle, whose empire covered all the earth, except Judæa alone. Both the one and the other, however, were actuated by a common animosity to the good principle, to whose throne they aspired, and they ambitiously endeavoured to reduce to vassalage all the souls of men, keeping them in a tedious and miserable captivity.

Another sect called themselves Cainites, from their veneration for the character of Cain, who, they asserted, was the offspring of a more potent energy, and therefore predominated over Abel, who sprang from a weaker origin. Others took the name of Judas Iscariot, and held that apostate in the highest reverence. Others rioted still more wildly in depravity and profaneness. Having, in our introductory remarks, presented the reader with the most prominent features of the Gnostic heresies in general, we shall merely repeat here (to account for the origin of those gems of which some of the most remarkable specimens have been reproduced) that it was one of their most remarkable tenets that malevolent spirits ruled the world, presided over universal nature, and caused all the diseases and sufferings of humanity. By knowledge or science, they believed, these spirits could be controlled, their power suspended, and even their malevolence charmed to the use and benefit of man. Of this science they boasted themselves the masters; and it consisted chiefly in the efficacy of numbers and of certain mysterious hieroglyphics and emblematic characters adopted chiefly from the Egyptians.

CHAPTER XV.

THE INDIAN RELIGIONS.—ANNOTATIONS ON THE SACRED WRITINGS OF THE HINDUS.

It is our design to institute a parallel between the theological Ideas of the Indian peoples and their Invaders and Conquerors, the Mahommedans, and the Philosophical Theses, stigmatised and rejected as Heresies, of the Neo-Platonists, or Half-Christians, or Mytho-Mystics —in fact, of the Gnostics. All the foregoing is intimately allied with the conclusions of the Rosicrucians, in as far as these varying speculators (the Gnostics and the other sects) were following out, although they occasionally branched off upon side roads, the *same objects* which are reputed to have been, ALREADY, in the hands of the Secret Brotherhood of The "Illuminated," or the Fraternity of the Red Cross.

The origin of the religious worship of the Hindus is lost in remote antiquity. All that has been handed down to us by oral tradition seems to confirm the hypothesis that for many ages anterior to the time of *Menu*, their first lawgiver, they were worshippers of one God only, whom they designated *Brühm Atma*, the "Breathing Soul," a spiritual Supreme Being, coeval with the formation of the world, without end, everlasting, permeating all space, the beneficent disposer of events. The worship of the Hindus at this period was probably simple, and their ceremonies were few. In process of time, however, the date of which cannot be correctly determined, they appear

N

to have adopted a material type or emblem of Brühm: a rude block of stone began to be set up. This was the *Phallus*, or, as they termed it, the LINGA. This emblem had reference to the procreative power seen throughout nature, and in that primæval age was regarded with the greatest awe and veneration. To the influence of this image was attributed the fructifying warmth which brought to perfection the fruits of the earth and contributed to the reproduction of man, animals, and everything that has life. This is the "deified attraction," or "magical coming together," of the Rosicrucians, and the deified "gravity" of the statistical or realising philosophers.

This simple and primitive idolatry came by degrees to diverge into the adoration of the element of Fire, and at length developed itself by institution of an emanation from *Brühm Atma*, or *Brähm Atma*, in his Triune capacity as Creator, Preserver or Saviour, and Destroyer. These attributes were deified under the names of *Brahma*, *Vishnu*, and *Siva*, on whom were conferred three *Gunas* or "Qualities"—viz., *Rajas* (passion), *Sat* (purity), and *Tumas* (darkness). This is the *Trimurti*. The word "*Trimurti*" means "three-formed," or "The Three." '*Murti* is to be taken as signifying also an image or likeness. Our vital souls are, according to the Védanta, no more than images of the Supreme Spirit. (*Asi. Res.*, vol. iii.)

The next step towards the formation of a Pantheon was the institution of *Avatas* and *Avantaras*—*i.e.*, greater and lesser Incarnations, by which one or other of the *Triad* imparted a portion of his divine essence both to men (generally Bahurdurs or heroes) and to brutes. The tendency to deify heroes and irrational creatures was not peculiar, however, to the Hindus, for the Assyrians, Etruscans, Greeks, and Romans had the same custom, as had also the Egyptians in a much more extended degree.

The system of *Avatas* was followed by an almost universal deification, not only of the elements and the heavenly bodies, but of every recognised attribute of the Supreme Being and of the Evil Spirit. Omnipotence, Beneficence, Virtue, Love, Vice, Anger, Murder, all received a tangible form, until at the present time the Hindu pantheon contains little short of a million Gods and Demi-Gods. It is admitted, however, that to many of them they pay only relative honour. It is a little remarkable that of this host of divinities, especially in Bengal, *Siva* is the God whom they are especially delighted to honour. As the Destroyer, and one who revels in cruelty and bloodshed, this terrible deity, who has not inaptly been compared to the Moloch of Scripture, of all their divinities suggests most our idea of the Devil. It may therefore be concluded that the most exalted notion of worship among the Hindus is a service of *Fear*. The *Brahmins* say that the other Gods are good and benevolent and will not hurt their creatures, but *Siva* is powerful and cruel, and that it is necessary to appease him.

Although this deity is sometimes represented in the human form in his images, it is not thus that he is most frequently adored. The most popular representation of him is unquestionably the *Linga*, a smooth stone rising out of another stone of finer texture, *similacrum membri virilis, et pudendum muliebre*. This emblem is identical with *Siva* in his capacity of " Lord of All."

It is necessary, however, to observe here that Professor Wilson, while admitting that "the *Linga* is perhaps the most ancient object of homage adopted in India," adds that it became popular "*subsequently to the ritual of the Vedhas*, which was chiefly, if not wholly, addressed to the Elements, and *particularly to Fire.*" How far the worship of the *Linga* is authorised by the Vedhas, Mr. Edward Sellon says, is doubtful.*

However this may be, it is abundantly clear that the *Lingaic*, or (which term covers the meaning generally) Phallic worship is the main purport of several of the *Puranas.*† Of this there cannot be a doubt.‡ The universality of Linga-Puja (or worship) at the period of the Mahommedan invasion of India, is well attested. The Idol destroyed by Mahmoud at Ghizni (notwithstanding the remarkable stories related by the Mahommedan chroniclers of a colossal image of human form which the Brahmins offered immense sums to save from destruction, and which, upon being shattered by a blow from Mahmoud's mace, disgorged a vast treasure of gold and precious stones of immense value, the whole of which story Wilson asserts is a pure fiction,) was nothing more than one of those mystical blocks of stone called Lingas. *Siva* under the type of the *Linga* is practically almost the only form in which that deity is reverenced. The prevalence of this worship throughout the whole tract of the Ganges, as far as Benares, is sufficiently conspicuous.

* In truth and in the abstract sense, it is precisely the same thing, only presented in another form. Phallic Worship is Fire-Worship.

† *Puranas*, the modern Scriptures of the Hindus, as distinguished from the Vedhas, or more ancient Scriptures.

‡ Wilson on Hindu sects (*As. Res.*, vol. xvii.)

In Bengal the *Lingam** Temples are commonly erected
in a range of six, eight, or twelve, on each side of a
Ghaut† leading to the river. Kalma is a circular group
of one hundred and eight temples erected by the Rajah
of Burdwan. These temples, and, indeed, all those found
in Bengal, consist of a simple chamber of a square form,
surmounted by a *pyramidal centre;* the area of each is
very small. The Linga of black or white marble, and
sometimes of alabaster slightly tinted and gilt, is placed
in the middle.

Speaking of *Siva* and Pawáti,‡ M. de Langlet says:—
" Les deux divinités dont il s'agit, sont très souvent et
très pieusement adorées sous la figure du Linga (le Phallus
des anciens) et de l'yoni dans leur mystérieuse conjunction. L'yoni se nomme *Bhaga* (*pudendum muliebre*),
Madheri douce, et *Argha*, vase en forme de bateau, dans
laquelle on offre des fleurs à la divinité; tels sont les noms
de *l'Adhera-Sacti* (energie de la conception vivifiée par le
Linga). Quand cette déesse est représentée par le
symbole que je viens d'indiquer, elle prend le nom de
Devi (divine), plus communément que ceux de *Bhavani*,
de Pracriti, &c. Suivant les théologiens Hindous, une
vive discussion s'éleva entre *Pawáti* (née des montagnes),

---

* The *Lin'gam*, or *Lingham* (with the *aspirate* H), is everywhere
the *protuberant*.

† Ghaut, "a high place," applied to a pass, such as the Laulpet
Pass, where travellers ascend from the campaign country to the table-
land of the Deccan ; also, and in this instance, signifying an artificial
"high place," constructed either of stone or marble, with an immense
flight of steps leading down to a river. There are numerous *ghauts* of
this description on the banks of the Ganges, where the banks are too
high to allow the people to approach the stream with safety.

‡ *As. Res.*, vol. xvii., pp. 208, 209, and 210.

et *Maha-deva* (le grand dieu), peu de temps après leur mariage, sur l'influence des sexes dans la production des êtres ; ils convinrent de créer séparément une race d'individus. Les enfants de *Maha-deva* furent nombreux, et se dévouèrent au culte de la *divinité mâle* ; mais ils manquaient d'intelligence et de force, et ils étaient mal conformés. Ceux de Pawáti étoient beaux, bien faits et d'un excellent naturel ; cependant, obsédés par les *Lingadja*, ou enfants de *Maha-deva*, ils envirent aux mains avec eux, et les vainquirent. *Maha-deva* allait dans sa fureur anéantir d'un coup d'œil les Yônîdja vainqueurs, si Pawáti ne l'eut appaisé. Les Brâhmanes offrent aux Linga des fleurs, et ont soin quand ils font leurs cérémonies d'allumer sept lampes, lesquelles selon Mathurin Veyssière la Croze, resemblent au chandelier à sept branches des Juifs,* qu'on voit à Rome sur l'arc de Titus. Les femmes portent des Lingas au cou et aux bras ; celles qui désirent devenir fecondes rendent à cette idole un culte tout particulier ; elles ont d'autant plus de confiance dans ses prêtres que ceux-ci font vœu de chastété."†

The offerings are presented at the threshold. Benares is the peculiar seat of this form of worship. The principal deity, Siva, there called Viweswarra, as observed already, is a Linga ; and most of the chief objects of pilgrimage are similar blocks of stone. No less than forty-seven Lingas are visited, all of pre-eminent sanctity ; but there are hundreds of inferior note still worshipped, and

---

* De Langlet is in error here. The *Punchaty,* as its name implies, consists of five, not seven, lamps.

† *Monuments Anciens et Modernes de l'Hindoustan,* par L. L. de Langlet. Paris : 2 vols., fol., 1810.

thousands whose fame and fashion have passed away. It is a singular fact, that upon this adoration of the pro-creative and sexual *Sacti* (or power) seen throughout nature, hinges the whole gist of Hindu faith, and not-withstanding all that has been said by half-informed per-sons to the contrary, this *puja* does not appear to be prejudicial to the morals of the people. "Among a people of such exuberant fancy as the Hindus," says Sir William Jones, "it is natural that everything should receive form and life. It is remarkable to what a degree their works of imagination are pervaded by the idea of sexuality.

"Indeed, it seems never to have entered into the heads of the Hindu legislators and people that anything natural could be offensively obscene, a singularity which pervades all their writings, but is no proof of the depravity of their morals; thence the worship of the *Linga* by the followers of *Siva*, of the *Yoni* by the followers of *Vishnu*." (*Sir William Jones's Works*, vol. ii., p. 311.) "It is unattended in Upper India by any indecent or indelicate ceremonies." (*Wilson on the Hindu Sects. As. Res.*, vol. xvii.)

We find amongst the sacred paintings of the Hindus numerous representations of devotees, both male and female, adoring the *Linga*; and a description of one of these pictures will suffice for all. The domestic temple, in which the emblem is usually placed, is a *dewal*, a term derived from *deva*, a deity, and *havela*, a house— *i.e.*, the "house of God." Indeed, the natives have no such word as "Pagoda" for their temples, which are always called *Dewals*.

The worshipper is seated, dressed, and arrayed in all her jewels, as directed by the ritual. In her right hand she holds a *mala,* or "rosary," of one hundred and eight round beads, which is not visible, as her hand is placed within a bag of gold brocade (*kampkab*), called *gumuki,* to keep off insects or any adverse influence. Her *langi,* or bodice, is yellow, her dress transparent muslin edged with gold (*upervastra*). In front of her are the five lamps, called *punchaty,* used in this *puja,* together with the *jari,* or spouted vessel, for lustral water; the *dippa,* or cup, to sprinkle the flowers which she has offered, and which are seen on the *Linga ;* and, lastly, the *gantha,* or sacred bell, used frequently during the recapitulation of the prescribed *muntras,* or incantations. Nearly all the *pujas* are conducted with frequent ringing of bells, the object of which is twofold, first to wake up the attention at particular parts of the service; and, secondly, to scare away malignant *dewas* and evil spirits; precisely, in fact, for the same reasons as they are used at the celebration of mass in Roman Catholic countries.

The Linga and the Earth are, according to the Hindus, identical, and the Mountain of Meru is termed the " Navel of the Earth." Meru is supposed to be the centre of the universe, and is said to be 8,400 *yojans* high, 32,000 broad at the top, 16,000 at the bottom. It is circular, and formed like an inverted cone. This notion was not confined to India, for when Cleanthes asserted that the earth was in the shape of a cone (*As. Res.,* viii.), this is to be understood only of this mountain, *Meru* of India. Anaximenes (*Plutarch de placit. philosoph.*) said that this column was plain and of stone, exactly like Meru—the *pargwette* (*Pawáti*) of the inhabitants of Ceylon (*Join-ville, As. Res.,* vol. vii.). " This mountain," says he, " is entirely of stone, 68,000 *yojanas* high, and 10,000 in circumference, and of the same size from the top to the bottom."

In India the followers of Buddha (*Trailoyeya-Derpana*) insist that that mountain is like a drum, with a swell in the middle, in that same form as the *tomtoms* used in the East. In the West the same opinion was expressed by Leucippus, and the *Buddhists* in India give that shape also to islands. This figure is given as an emblem of the reunion of the powers of Nature. *Meru* is the sacred and primæval *Linga :* and the earth beneath is the mysterious *Yoni* expanded, and open like the *Padma* or Lotus. The convexity in the centre is the navel of *Vishnu*, and the physiological mysteries of their religion are often represented by the emblem of the Lotus; where the whole flower signifies both the earth and the two principles of its fecundation. The germ is both *Meru* and the *Linga;* the petals and filaments are the mountains which encircle *Meru*, and are also the type of the *Yoni*. The four leaves of the *calix* are the four vast regions turning towards the four cardinal points. Of the two geographical systems of the Hindus, the first or more ancient (as set forth in the *Puranas*) describes the Earth as a convex surface gradually sloping towards the borders, and surrounded by the ocean. The second, and more modern system, is that which has been adopted by their astronomers. The followers of the *Puranas* consider the earth as a *flat surface*, or nearly so, and their knowledge does not extend much beyond the old continent, or the superior hemisphere.

The leaves of the Lotus represent the different islands in the ocean around *Jambu*, and, according to the Hindu system, the whole earth floats upon the waters like a boat.

The *Argha** of the Hindus and the cymbium of the Egyptians are also emblems of the earth, and of the *Yoni*. The *Argha* or Cymbium signifies a vessel, cup or dish, in which fruits or flowers are offered to the Deities, and ought to be in the shape of a boat; though many are oval, circular, or even square.

Iswarra, or Bacchus, is styled *Argha-Nautha*, or " Lord," the original contriver of the " boat-shaped vessel;" and *Osiris* the *Iswarra*, or Bacchus of Egypt, according to Plutarch, was commander of the *Argo*, and was represented, by the Egyptians, in a boat, carried on the shoulders of a great many men. The ship worshipped by the *Suevi*, according to Tacitus, was the *Argha*, or *Argo*, the type of the *pudendum muliebre*. The *Argha*, or *Yoni*, with the *Linga* of stone, is to be found all over India as an object of worship. Flowers are offered to it,

---

* The three words *Amba*, *Nabbi*, and *Argha* seem to have caused great confusion among the Greek mythologists, who even ascribe to the earth all the fanciful shapes of the *Argha*, which was intended at first as a mere emblem. Hence they represented it in the form of a boat, of a cup, or of a quoit with a boss in the centre, sloping towards the circumference, where they placed the ocean.—*Agathem.*, book i., c. i. Others describe the earth as a square or parallelogram, and Greece was supposed to lie on the summit, with Delphi in the navel, or central part of the whole.—*Pind. Pyth.* 6. *Eurip. Ion.*, v. 233. The Jews, and even the early Christians, insisted that the true navel of the earth was *Jerusalem*, and the Mohammedans, *Mecca*. The Argha is a type of the *Adhera-Sacti*, or Power of Conception, exerted and vivified by the Linga or Phallus, one and the same with the ship Argo, which was built, according to Orpheus, by Juno and Pallas, and according to Apollonius, by Pallas and Argos, at the instance of Juno.— *Orph. Argon.* v., 66. *Apoll.*, lib. ii., 5, 1190. *As. Res.*, vol. iii.

and the water, which is poured on the *Linga*, runs into the rim which represents the Yoni, and also the *fossa navicularis*, and *Iswarra* is sometimes represented standing instead of the Linga in the middle, as Osiris in Egypt. (*As. Res.*, viii.)

Plutarch has said of the Egyptians, that they had inserted nothing into their worship without a reason. " Nothing merely fabulous is introduced, nothing superstitious, as many suppose; but their institutions have either a reference to morals or to something useful in life." The mass of mankind lost sight, however, of morality in the multiplicity of rites, as it is easier to practise ceremonies than to subdue passions; so it was in India and Egypt.

In the course of investigating the ceremonies of the Hindus, and in attempting to elucidate their meaning, it will be found necessary to draw an analogy between them and those of the Egyptians. The resemblance is very striking; they mutually serve to explain each other. When the Sepoys, who accompanied Lord Hutchinson in his Egyptian expedition, saw the temple at Denderah, they were very indignant with the natives of the place for allowing it to fall into decay, conceiving it to be the temple of the consort of their own god, Siva; a fact, to say the least of it, no less singular than interesting. The religion of Egypt no doubt had its origin in India.

The annihilation of the sect and worship of *Brahma*, as the *Iswarra* or "Supreme Lord," is described at large in the *Kasichandra* of the *Scanda-Puran;* where the three powers are mentioned as contending for precedence. *Vishnu* at last acknowledges the superiority of Siva; but *Brahma*, on account of his presumptuous obstinacy, had one of his heads cut off by Siva, and his *puja*, or worship, was abolished.

The intent of this legend is evidently to advance the claims of the *Siva* sect; and if we substitute the contending facts for the battle of the *Deutas*, or angels, the fable will appear not quite destitute of historical fact, nor wholly without foundation.

CHAPTER XVI.

MYSTIC ANATOMY, AND THE MASTER PASSION OR "THE ACT."

THESE sections of our book are drawn from considerations arising out of the mysterious philosophy of the
inter-celestial and terrestrial human anatomy of the experts of the ancient classic times and of the middle ages,
and particularly from the remote myths and mythologies
of the Oriental countries.

The whole system and the view of the act, both
theoretic and practical, is considered, whether it be viewed
as a rite, a sacrifice, a sacrament, a magic spell or practice, and is developed and commented upon according to
the mystic doctrines propounded by Jacob Bœhm. The
examination of this difficult and evading subject is de-
duced according to the mystical ideas outlined in origin
and regularity as produced out of the occult influence of
the planets in genuine Chaldaic and authoritative astrology,
which, totally misunderstood, are blundered and spoiled in
modern attempted renderings (which in themselves supply
their own proof of insufficiency, and are their own confuta-
tion), and in the hints and suggestions gathered from amidst
the mazes which are purposely interwoven to blunt and to
lead away, to disappoint, and to baffle inquiry, of the
Cabala, in which all the learning and knowledge of the
old world was shut up, and its power and light laid aside
when the Old Primæval World was "Ruined." The
action, inter-action, and cross-action of the stars in the
mutual effects and operation upon each other, of the

planets, and more particularly the cross-moving and the amplifying and waning, crescent and decrescent powers (aggressive and defensive) of the Moon—all relatively qualifying and harmonising—all this is the telluric and celestial history, " set, as it were, to sleep" in the divine " orchestration," springing to life, meaning, and vigour in the " music of the spheres" (no false thing, but a real thing), by means of which the ministers of the originating God made the creation of the World possible— Nature, in this super-essentially divine handiwork, finding at once its support and its imperfections in the reluctant, persistently protesting " bass," without which contrast music would be impossible. Music, in other senses than those of man—who, in reality (as he has become in his lost and depraved state), is " deaf as an adder"—is the " air of Paradise." Sometimes, even now, at magic moments, with those who are gifted to apprehend its effect, there come floating over the soul dim, dreamy recollections of that happy place, mingled with sad reflective consciousness, that, through the treason of his great progenitor, Adam, man has for ever lost his first-intended, celestial home.

The doctrine of the mystics is that the Second Great Luminary, the mighty Moon (ruler and Queen of the Darkness), is all-powerful in certain senses. She takes half-part in the rendering of men's fate. She labours (in the half-part) to make up the human and every creature's destiny. The figure of the Man, like a phantom, has to pass through " Mansions"—or the thirteen lunations—in the year. Man is made " in the moon," for the mystic passage of the child in the mother's womb is marked by distinct stages at these nine strange gates (or more properly ten) through which the child passes to birth, or to the true moment for the deciding horoscope in astrology, when the child, for the first time, confronts the stars. The influences of the moon are feminine influences, and refer to the secondary or responsive principle, pulsative throughout nature, as constituted now in the material formularies. We can alone find the life and the vigour and the purpose and meaning of music, as detailed in its intertangling effects and dominating play upon the affections and passions in its hieroglyphic musical telegraphics. These are operating upon the sensitive nerves, and the heart of man—as we witness every day when the administration of the music is prosperous and adequate—in the swelling and sinking of this sympathetic communication passing between the soul of man and the divinities.

We may now consider the mystic physiology of the human being ("Male and Female created He them") and the *rationale* (celestial and otherwise) of the methods and the motives and purposes of Generation. This we will recommend and desire as not to be perused except with a raised mind and in a serious spirit—in a word, we would be understood to wish that all who do not feel themselves capable of this philosophical coolness and reticence, and of this abstract mode of study, and of this critical seriousness, should forego this important section. The whole subject is sought to be raised into high, abstract and spiritual levels, and the topics are reduced into narrow definitions. Lurking principles in the physiology of the " human construction" are examined with care. The range of statements springs from out the profound mystic anatomical philosophy of those masters of speculation,

Henry Cornelius Agrippa, Albertus Magnus, Plato, and the Idealists; Battista Van Helmont, Guglielmus Postellus, Jerome Cardan, and the Mystics; Robertus de Fluctibus, and the Alchemists; Jacob Bœhm, and the Transcendentalists;—all the greatest minds of antiquity and of the middle ages.

Coition, human, is synthesis—it is the union of "Half-Sex," Man (so assumed in this abstract sense), and "Half-Sex," Woman (so assumed, also, in this abstract sense). The union of these "Two" half-sexes is the establishment of a "Whole" Sex—hermaphrodite (Hermes-Aphrodite, Venus-Mercury). The mechanical definition of Sex is power of blissful protrusion, human organic shooting, willed, conscious magnetism (for an end), with climax of dissolution and destruction (in the end), perishing as in the "flower" of this "stalk." Thus Cornelius Agrippa and Paracelsus—thus the mystic anatomists, like Fludd and Van Helmont.

The orders "increase" and "multiply" are orders to be taken as identical, although, in fact, they are directly contradictory. It is these things which are set against each other which constitute the stupendous and irresistible natural temptation (obtained out of shame, cr out of denial and disgrace,) of all this enchanted side of life.

It is from these conjoint reasons that, in its mystery, the universal success and universal power of this side of life springs. It is inseparable from the human being, and yet, strange to say, in the philosophic, and therefore the true, sense, it is only accidental to the human being. This passion is the master passion. This passion is the key-note of everything. All the other passions are made the servants of this dominant one. Ambition is made a fool by it. Revenge mainly is caused by it. Love rage is worst rage. Avarice pours out its treasure to obtain it. Pride submits the lowest to it. Luxury is the greatest in it.

Therefore, for these reasons, which are indisputable (as all the world and the experience of all the world witnesses), both in the past time and in the present, there is the greater necessity that out of man's responsible nature (for he has a responsible nature, from fear in regard to himself,) should be derived the natural safeguards against this endowment or the reverse? (as which shall we distinguish it?). As we well know, all the grace, beauty, delight, and glory of life spring from it, as well as the possibility of horror and terror. It is a heaven on earth in some senses, and yet, in its very nature, there is a possibility of converting this heaven into a hell. In any way, it is a heaven which resigns all its flames (bright flames) of joy, and leaves (in the end) in our hands only these natural physical results of combustion, dust—the mortal residuum which perpetuates the heirship of degradation and of shame. Man is the heir of the first Adam, and therefore he is born into disgrace and has consequently to face the penalty, for the pure angels avert from him.

"Cursed now is the ground for thy sake." Who shall save him, this ruin of ruins, this "Man," out of the terror of the abyss into which he has fallen through the treason of his first progenitor, yielding in his weakness to the lures of the Great Enemy? Who shall rescue the condemned? Only the pitying Champion whose Immortal Mercy has traversed all the worlds, bad as well as good. We instance this to show

that the idea of the Saviour is an inseparable necessity for
fallen Man. We think that the world is wrong in its
thus childishly ignoring the philosophical and critical
examination of this all-important range of objects of
attention, which we feel soliciting and provocative in our
body every day of our lives, and without the regulated
indulgence of which, as the chief spur, we should wither,
spoil, and consume. These are things which must be
thought of, whether we will or no. There is a prudery—
which, after all, is only hypocrisy—which is worse
than the reasons for shame or the exhibition and the
confession of even the shame itself. Nature has no
shames. But the human creature, in his humanity, has
shames—overpowering, ineradicable shames.

While Man remains Man it is impossible to resist the
force of his natural desires, which we do not see why we
should not designate by their true, well-understood name,
lust. There is an irresistible rush to the Female, beautiful
body. There is a certain sort of wild, ungovernable impulse, totally beyond reason and sense, exhibited in all these
successful cases, which we shall not be far wrong in characterising as a kind of the wreaking of a feeling, similar to
"rage," however absurd the expression may seem, upon this
presented personality. Against all the mischiefs, dangers,
and inconveniences which would be sure to arise from the
mistimed presentment of this irresistibly beautiful shape,
man has taken his measures from the beginning of time.
Thence dress. Thence (particularly) the female dress,
artfully contrived, in all judicious, well-regulated countries,
to disappoint, to evade, to mask, to involve, to abnegate,
to conceal. Thence "skirts"—the longer the better in
the puritanic sense,—the fuller, the wider, in the (neces-

sary, in society) defrauding sense. Therefore we cover woman's beautiful body carefully up. Thence the long robe and the hiding of the legs of woman.* Hence the

* It has been a question with the mystic anatomists, and with artists who have made progress in refinement and in occultism, whether the beauty of the outlines of the *legs* of women—strangely as such a theory may sound—has not been greatly contributed to, really, by *exposure*, and that the covering them up (in the long robe) has not conduced to their shapely *languishment.* This may partly arise (indeed, we think it *does* arise) from the natural self-consciousness of women, and from their sensitiveness when disrobed. For nature is most artful in its address to the senses. This mystic, natural heightening of the gracefulness of the shape of the female lower limbs, may also originate in the magnetism springing between woman's eager response (sanctified by nature) and man's sexual poetical desires, in the high artistic, mythological sense. This is a strange philosophy ; but it boasts fullest authority in some of the Rosicrucian profundities, even although these latter may not be of earth, but may spring from magic, though they seem to bear such intimate reference to it. From a consideration of the above reasons, it is clearly in the interest of women to wish to inspire intense personal desire for their charms in the minds of men ; and, to secure the success of this paramount intention, it must naturally be their aim (if they were allowed) to freely display their legs, the beauty of these latter being still more important—strangely to say—even than their faces as the incitement in the great end of woman. Thus it is the policy of women (and the sharpest-minded among them know it) to show as much as possible of their lower limbs, this disclosure being the chief means of exciting that passion (the most flattering and charming to woman) in which lieth the power to make the greatest fools of men (even of the wisest, as all history, sacred and profane, avoucheth)—certainly of *all* men. Men, in fact, by nature, have been made the slaves of women, in some respects. From some of these reasons arise the results which prove the power, even the enthusiasm, of their mystic sacredness, of carnivals and masquerades (all "saturnalia" of their kind), where the sexes interchange dress and characteristics, and women become as men and men become as women. Thence mimes, mimics, grotesques, saltimbanques—those that the French call *folles, folletins, débardeurs* and *débardeuses,* and all the infinite variety of that fantastical, natural and unnatural "pied populace," with Momus and the mopes, Satan and the

universal anonymity of the lower half of the person of woman, which in reality is an extinguishment biblically "for the fear of her." We have Scripture warrant for this fear in the ordinances of the Bible. Women are commanded to "cover their heads" in that obscure text and in that strange deterrent warning, for "fear of the angels." There is a vast amount of magic mysticism mingling with these special orders in regard to women in the sacred Scriptures which we do not elect—at all events

satyrs and the sylvans, and the representatives and the caricatures of that playful "Father" and "Mother" of "Nature"—animate and reanimate, natural and supernatural—who presided at (and joined in) that grand carnival and display, and "gran" Biblical "*festa*," when the multitude of the Children of Israel, finding that Moses delayed his coming down from the Mountain (of Sinai), dissatisfied with their chiefs, rose in rebellion to demand of Aaron a visible trophy, or talisman, or supernatural object, or god, "to go before them." And when their desire was acceded to, they bowed down before the Golden Calf, and in their crowds they ran riot, in a sort of frantic, sacred defiance, and "Ate and drank, and rose up to *play*." As to this "*play*"— what it was—and what was its universal character—and that it was, in fact, a grand, indecent orgie—all keen-sighted antiquarians and Bible explorers and explainers (all, of course, except the rigidly orthodox) are now fully agreed. This "god," to "go before them," the grand talisman to incite them to victory, was undoubtedly the Phallus, demanded by the Israelites in their recollection of the mysteries of the Egyptians. For the "sign" of the *phallus* (*phallos*, φαλλος, in the Greek) is in the hand of all the innumerable figures, lavished with an overpoweringly majestic, enforcing reiteration on every flat surface, and upon every column and mighty frieze all over the wilderness, as it may be called, of the sand-engulphed structures and myriad monuments of ancient Egypt—unread (or wholly misread) as this wonderful symbol has hitherto been. It has been ignored, or turned away from (perhaps properly and laudably) through all the latter ages. But all the above will prove the universality of this Phallic religion. It will also show the ignorance of the ages in regard to it, and the thickheaded prudery of the moderns in their thinking it a shameful instead of a noble sign.

in this present place—to refer to, certainly not more explicitly to explain. In certain senses a beautiful, perfectly-formed naked woman is—singular and unexpected as the expression may seem until the appreciation realises the reasons—a terrible object, we mean in the sense—the abstract sense—of awe at her as a wonder, as the work of a Maker, and as the presentation of her as a temptation. Thus we see how a naked woman may be terrible because she is an awful object, possibly because of her almost impossibly to be resisted charms, by reason that when she is in this nude condition she constitutes the most dangerous of all temptations. And when not vulgarised by the world's ways and ideas and contact, by the indignities which are to be found in nature (and which nature yet insists upon)—a woman thus disclosed, we repeat, is perfect, and is a phenomenon, an Ideal, a perilous presentment from " we know not whence," designed, begotten, or gifted ! She is an ideal, contemplated, as it were, under impossible, or, rather, under seemingly treasonable conditions, and the most magnificent phenomenon, or (in this abstract, transcendental sense) unintelligible object which the world (not this world only, which is nothing, but the supersensual world, the world of the angels and devils,) has seen. The lower half of the person of woman, from the waist downwards, is sacred. Beauty—" wreaking" and " wrecking" the desiring one upon it—beauty, whether male or female, for it is either, although the beauty that attracts sensually must be of the feminine order, for strength is the characteristic of man, while beauty is the condition of justification in the characteristics of the woman,—beauty, we repeat, in its lure, is a magnet to

the human nature. It is all-subduing—there is no limit
to its power. It needs most carefully to be guarded
against. The wise person should always continually and
carefully watch himself (or herself). For passion—fierce
passion—is frequently alike the lot with both sexes.
This surmounting fact presses up to recognition in all
time and from a thousand histories. It is strange that
women should entertain a passion for their own sex, but,
nevertheless, it is true, although they have no power to
produce direct pleasure with each other. Particularly is
it true with those women who, from natural constitution,
are most prone to self-indulgence; and still more singularly with that luxurious class called ladies of pleasure,
who enjoy the most liberal opportunities, from the regular
exercise of their profession, in the expected and in the
properly conceded way. But a perverted and a pampered
imagination is full of tricks. We find this irregularity
with all the appetites, which, in truth, require the most
careful government and a most despotically-applied discipline. It is well known that among courtesans, particularly in France and Italy and in South America, some
of the most rapturous engrossments, of this passionate,
particular kind, exist between women, mutually in love,
in the sensual respect (yes, and in the sentimental respects,
too) with each other, and giving way to this love with
an abandonment far exceeding their attachment to men.
There is much of this referred to in many old French
books, notably in the celebrated memoirs of Brantôme.
Two women have been known to form a very faithful
league for pleasing each other. Some women of a
peculiarly sensitive, even highly refined character, as
well as others more irregularly and defiantly disposed,

have been known to disdain, disregard, and even to
hate the approach of men, and to lavish all their liking
upon women ; or, if retaining any preference for men,
regarding those most fondly who most closely resembled
the alluring external characteristics of their own elegant
sex, so far as curving lines and lineaments were concerned.
This disdain and dislike even of men likely apparently to
please them, is a curious characteristic of the volatile and
uncertain sex, in regard of whom nothing can be fixed
but instability. No man can in reality know what is
passing in a woman's mind, even when she is looking,
with apparently the most serious attention, at him, particularly if she be young and attractive and fortified by
the knowledge gained by experience that she is beautiful
and that she has charms. Instances have been known—
indeed, it is there that they are chiefly prevalent—among
the Phrynes and Aspasias, both of old days and of
modern times, of the most decided preference of women
(by women) over men for infatuation for this fond
companionship,* and for intercourse in irregular respects.

---

* It is curious that men, at least most men, do not feel any jealousy
(or, if jealousy, it is remote) for this kind of thing. When they would
be excited to the utmost extremities of jealousy at the idea of a male—
whether man or boy—being thus situated in regard to a woman for
whom they may entertain a passion, there is no special movement in the
mind when the rival is a female only—almost to whatever lengths the
partiality may be carried. This may partly arise (besides from the man's
knowing that the woman can never fully succeed) from the man's
experiencing—in a sly sense—a feeling of relief from his responsibility,
and from his secret satisfaction at the " relief guard" being established,
in his interest, in the matter of the duties naturally continuously due, and
expected of him, notwithstanding the advanced time of life to which he
may have (happily) attained. It is quite a mistake to suppose that youth
is important in this respect, in the exercise of certain powers. Every-

Desire, in these regards, with women as well as with men,—and more particularly with women on account of the feebleness and the lavish warmth and fantastic impressionability of their nature—is most eccentric. It is never to be estimated, or, indeed, provided against. It baffles reason. It is contrary, sometimes, to common sense. It will fly in the face (as far as it dares) of the most ordinary ideas of decency. Shall we be taken wrongly (admiring women as we do) in asserting that, as a rule and in the fundamental comparison of the real radical natures of the two sexes, men are more modest than women? It sounds very extraordinary. We do not mean otherwise than properly to put this impression forward. We do not imply this as an imputation, but in the sense of nearness to nature, like the instincts of children. The idea of the loveable male is not the rough, hirsute Hercules-like, or Neptune-like (*Poseidon*), or even Mars-like champion-man, but the Hylas, the Hyperion, the Apollo, the Adonis, the Ganymede, the Narcissus, the Hermaphroditus,—the ideal being, or demi-divinity, truly the something resembling a god, but not quite like it, the creature whose charms and seductive, slender graces more closely resemble the insinuating attractions of woman's own magical sex. The proofs of this assertion are sufficiently abundant. The most masterful passion ever entertained, notably in the instance of a

thing depends upon the mind, and upon the firm state and the elasticity of the nervous system. It is our decidedly firm opinion—formed from observations of a large range—that continual smoking, particularly in the early part of the day, and the too habitual use of intoxicating fluids and similar methods of excitement, beyond being generally and permanently injurious to men, are compromising and enfeebling in the foregoing very important private respect.

woman possessed of so much and such unbounded power, when everything real and physical, in this respect, lay at her feet, was that fiery and yet most tender love—the most persistent and permanent of all her passions, it is said—entertained by the Imperial sovereign of Russia, the Empress Catherine the Second, to whom was applied the rarest and yet certainly the most distinguished possible title in this very grand, in one sense, and yet very irregular and disturbing in another sense—we mean the degradation or the dignity—which shall we call it? or, rather, may we not call it "both in one," and "one in both," being distinguished as "La più futatrice nel mondo?" And this is the fierce, and yet the softest love —which is said to have been entertained by this tremendous woman—as merciless in her cruelties as in her lusts, for a little slip of a man (much more like a woman than a man), with flowing ringlets, the whitest of skins, and the smallest and most delicate of features,—"the fair-faced Lanskoi," as Byron calls him. Catherine is said to have grieved terribly for him after his death, and to have shut herself up for a week after being apprised of it, giving way to a passion of tears, refusing to see anybody, and forgetful altogether of the cares of State—nay, of everything which would distract her attention for one moment from the regret and affliction which possessed her for the loss of her (at once) toy and favourite. This is the effeminate style of man which some say—and we are inclined to believe that they have reason for what they say—exercises the greatest power, though it is never acknowledged and is always denied, over female fancies. Lord Byron asserts, in his "Don Juan," that this is the kind of "male-female" semblance which is very dangerous in its rivalries to the more manly type, and he speaks of it with an affirmative sort of poetic *nonchalance* as

> "That fond, Parisian aspect which upset old Troy,
> And founded Doctors' Commons."

Beauty, we repeat, in its lure is a magnet to the human nature. Man must cease to be man or be turned into a stock to withstand it. Love's very torment, and writhing of forceful impatience at it, in the act of generation, has been converted by Nature into all-conquering, but mad and unintelligible joy, wreaking a "heaven of sense," as it seems. The pudenda, both in the male and the female, are magnets, and their natural, deliriously delightful presentment to each other is magic-magnetism, superadded and "incidental" only (let it be remarked) to man's first nature. These phenomenal organs—superb and miraculous in their special address or use—are "Positive-Negative" in Man, "Negative-Positive" in Woman. Woman is "Man," halfway forward. Man is "Woman," halfway backward. Both are corporeally and sexually One, in complete coition, or double-tie, or identification of "two singles," into temporary, absolute "one single." Man—sharp, acute, and piercing forward: woman—blunt and receptive in a passionately eager abyss, gaping (to use an ugly word, we admit, concerning it) into magic joy, backward. But that which meets and conflicts is the same passionate battle with each against each, seeking selfish victory, and finding victory in defeat and disgrace, defeat in which all joy falls to the earth again in its accomplishment and shame. Hence the sacredness, mystery, and miracle of the "act" (which is worship of its kind, and the greatest worship of its kind), and hence the horrible sin of misacting, or misreading, or reversing the purposes of Nature in the indulgence of this act through unnatural means and with unnatural objects, which implies the "supernatural cancer," branded with the curse of God in all physiology, in all religions, in all beliefs, in all natural facts and results. Hence are these implied sins more than sins—they are guilt, and treason, and horror against the "universal" nature, corporeal and spiritual. They are treasons abhorrent against spirit. Thus this—rightly looked at—awful act secures and perpetuates disease. And its withholding also secures and perpetuates disease, in grand contradiction to life. This is the contradictory balance that holds Nature at bay.

Love's very torment and writhing in the act of generation is—in the mystic and abstract sense—a penitential sacrifice (it is, as one class of the Gnostics say, an offering to and acknowledgment of the sovereignty of the Sinister, or Evil Genius, who holds, mystically and mythically, the one half of the balance of the post-diluvian "Zodiac"—at once the seat of the Olympus of the gods, in the one half, and the Tartarus, or the nether end of the immortal spiritual cosmography and cosmogony, in the other—when the original "Ecliptic," or cross band, or long-protracted, in man's measures (or instantaneously effected, in God's measures), path of conflict, or traverse of the angelic combative "Battle-Field," changed, or expanded, or opened out (or widened) from the original "Ten Signs," or ten stages of "Creation," to the latter "Twelve Signs," or "Twelve Processes" of reconciled, or (conditionally) pardoned, "Creation." All this is necessarily very obscure; indeed, to ordinary senses and ordinary means of interpretation it is unintelligible, but it is so only according to the ordinary world's method, or to the scholastic methods of acceptance, which the cabalistic experts wholly reject as mistaken, and hold in utter scorn. The cabalistic philosophers contend that they alone hold the keys—necessarily in the most secret and jealous (and of course effectual) guardianship—which unlock all the mysteries of time, space, and eternity, and of Heaven and Hell, and all the wonders of the inexhaustible physical universe. Hence the importance of the Phallic doctrines and of the magic validity of the Phallic religion, since these only can be esteemed declarative of the purposes of God and of the meaning of the production of all things—mortal and spiritual both—into this prodigious and portentous universe—truly prodigious, as all men know; truly portentous, as the chosen ones, or the enlightened ones, are convinced.

But to return to our Phallic theme. The act of generation has been converted, even in its frenzied pain and in its painful frenzy, into an all-conquering but mad and unintelligible joy,—a wreaking as into a " heaven of sense," as it seems, of which, metaphorically and ideally,—for figures and metaphors express real things after all, and things real in the world, as prophecies, and as a sort of prophetical adumbration, so to call the sort of thing not yet acted in the world, or not yet come to pass (although, in all certainty, coming to pass), things—that is, events and incidents—sometimes trivial, sometimes important, that rest or linger in the limbo or mists of possibility, or that may be either hurried or retarded, or even effaced or changed, as may accord with the superhuman and supernatural counsels of the invisible Rulers and Guides, filling that unknown and unimagined world of which these mysterious visionary *disjecta membra* are the objects. Thus prophecies and prefigurings may be true in the sense that now it is not yet time that has arrived to us, although it be the time that is past, to the intelligencies which "at once can look both backward and forward." Now, to God there can be no such thing as time, because the future is as much past to him as the past is already past to us. And we know that if we project the farthest from our view the "abysses of time" all becomes as unknown, as untrue, and as much mist and vapour as the very future, as the very morrow, as the nearest, even as the very next hour, to any given moment.

Thus prophecies of things not yet acted are yet true of the things to be acted, as the future is already the past in the Mind of the Divine. Because God is the " whole that is."

The mistake of those who will refuse to raise their minds to understand mysterious subjects connected with religion would be provoking were it not pitiable. For the want of the power of imaginative self-raising, which is produced only out of enthusiasm—which, of course, is set against common sense—the whole story of the " Holy Grael," which means the mystic body of the Lord Jesus Christ, the mysteries of the " Round Table," of the " Holy Eucharist," as understood in the Roman Catholic and Greek Churches, the life and career of King Arthur, and the achievements—romantic and traditionary as they were—of the Knights of that wondrous Court which displayed its chivalric and majestic shows at Caerleon, at Camelot, and in cities as gloriously romantic and poetically defunct as cities in clouds, the adventures of the

Knights Errant and the Twelve Paladins of the great
Emperor Charlemagne; nay, the deeply touching and
magnanimous account of the foundation of the "Most
Noble Order of the Garter," with its glorious warlike
meanings—abstruse and mystical as they are—all these
go for nothing in these days. They are reckoned out-
worn, superseded, merely fanciful, regarded as nothing—
that is, reckoned nothing of importance—in the general
mind—even the highest educated—we mean academically
instructed—general mind. All these great matters of
thought, all such stories and ideas, the Sagas of the
Nibelungen—the Scandinavian Pantheon, filled as it is
with gods and heroes,—legends, history—all that can
instruct, delight, and elevate, if it cannot be reconciled to
the hardest, most commonplace, even vulgar common
sense, or cannot be found to be of real literal, pro-
ducible use in some way or other, is undervalued and
passed over with contemptuous neglect, if not actually
derided.

In the grand supernatural contention of which we have
the tradition only, the mythic "Red Dragon," which
means the one half of the whole circle of things, is a
Master against whom, and with whom, the never-ending
(until the "New Jerusalem") war is waged, the "angelic
war." It is the "Child Chivalry," otherwise the "Innocence and the Power," which is to conquer. Child-
chivalry is a word little likely to be understood by a
reader fortified only in the knowledge of the colleges
and schools; and yet that word and the idea of the
"Innocence" and the "Power," lie at the foundation of
all the Christian theosophy. Childhood of valour (meaning its simplicity), Maidhood of valour (meaning its

purity),* are the characteristics of the *beau-idéal* of the Champion—of the Knights Errant—of the Brothers of the Holy Graël. The sword in the right hand of this mythic Champion, the "sworn one" of the Red Cross of the Crucifixion, the "sworn one" of the "Crucified" (of course feminine in this regard), "Rose," Saint Michael in heaven—the generalissimo and commander-in-chief of the armies of God, known as the Patron Saint of England, in his innocently white field, as depicted and emblazoned by the augurs or heralds, the natural high priests and hierophants of the myths and mysteries,

* This passage is significant in the sense of the champion, strong in his weakness, strong in the strength of his humility, that is, weakness in his dependency, or vacuity, as the fit receptacle for the pouring in of the Spirit of God, or possession by the Celestial Spirit, or by the Holy Ghost; which, of course, only expresses a purely spiritual idea. Such was David, the shepherd boy, the favourite of the Lord, the chosen of the Lord. Such were all the powerful "child champions," or "virgin champions"—strong in the might of the Lord, in their incapacity for pollution, in their invincible purity as saints. Such was Joan of Arc among the women. Judith and Jael were champion women of, perhaps, another stamp; but they became holy women in the offering up and in the sacrifice of their bodies, which, perhaps, both did gloriously, the one in the instance of Sisera, the other in the instance of Holofernes, for the magnificent object of the saving of their people—which was the acceptance by God of their saintship—the lesser reasons giving way to, and emerging in, the greater, and the "end" sanctifying and justifying the "means."

Another exemplification of this idea of the "Child-Champion," or the spotless and sinless and unconscious "Child of God," or "Cherub," in the youthful and mature sense, not in the childish sense (child-*like*, not childish), may be found in the lines—referring to the "model soldier," as incapable of vaunt or self-value as he is incapable of fear, even in the roar of battle and in presence of a thousand deaths—

"Of boasting, more than of a bomb afraid,
A soldier should be modest as a maid."

and the proper interpreters of all such—that sword of Saint Michael, or of the Champion of Heaven, or sword of Solomon,* the King of Israel and the Enchanter, who

* "The Sword of 'Solomon, the King of Israel,' or 'The Enchanter.'" It is exceedingly curious how these mysterious ideas have found their exemplification in the forms of heraldry, which, in its origin, · was a sacred science. Through heraldry and its powers of range over symbolism—which are perfect of their kind—the mysteries of religion were promulgated. The scientific details of heraldry, besides being eminently picturesque, are full of purpose and of symbolical richness. From this myth of the "sword" of Solomon, the King of Israel, and the Wizard; or the "Gladius" of the Archangel Saint Michael (the "Tyler" and the "Sentinel" of "Heaven"—taken as the "Lodge," in the Masonic sense), and the piercing spear, or the gladius or sword of Saint George, and its miraculous operation and prophetic effect in the striking through of the "throat" of the "Dragon,"—through these strangely abstruse, metaphysical notions, arises the Gnostic idea of the "second interference of God" with his creation, through his chief declarant, as combatant minister,—Saint Michael, "armed with his thunder," who is represented (refer to the Apocalypse) as traversing the "worlds visible and invisible." In regard of this great mystery arises to recognition the "cleft" of the Imperial diadem of the sovereigns of Russia. Over the "cleft" rises the magnificently jewelled signal of redemption—the "Cross." The Emperor of Russia is the Czar, Csar, or Cæsar—that is, the Cæsar, or Kaiser, or Kæsar (the letters C and K are convertible),—the Emperor (the successor of Constantine) of the East, when the Imperial Eagle of Rome became "double-headed." The Cæsar or Emperor, both of the East and of the West, is also, in the senses derived from the Orientals, in the Ishmaelitish, or "Left-Handed" acceptation—for an explanation of which refer to other parts of this book, or to "The Rosicrucians," Second Edition, London, 1879—the "Houssa," "Uzza," "Huzza," "Uss," or "Huss" (with a sexless meaning), or the Magical Son, or "Child" of the Woman, he who, in guise (or disguise) of the "Prince," sitteth at the "right hand" of Supreme Regality, "until his enemies are made his footstool," or until the left-handed side of Creation is vanquished or re-arranged. The Emperor of Germany is, at this period, the second Cæsar or Emperor—that is, the Emperor of the West—the legitimate successor of Charlemagne, though it is a dis-

has fastened the Devil down in the abyss, and placed his seal upon him (the pentagon, in magic) that tremendous sign, known in magic story by the name of the "Wizard's Foot"—that triumphant glaive has passed sheer through the "Wilds of Hell" and has cloven it (metaphorically) in half. All this is rhapsodical, of course, but it is the informing spirit of the Apocalypse and of the prophecies. It vivifies and insinuates, like a thread of fire, through all

puted point who is, or ought to be, this Emperor properly, among the heralds, whether it should be rightly the Emperor of Germany, sprung from the "Bo-Russi," or "Po-Russi," or the "Prussian" (B and P also, let it be remarked, are convertible letters in the dialects). The syllable "Bo," or "Po," is originally Taurine—the same is to be remarked of the pre-syllable "Bo"—in the name of the country, *Bo*hemia, all this intimating the early *Bovine* or *Taurine*, mythic, magic descent of these Northern Bovine (or Taurine) barbarous hordes. The supporters of the Royal Prussian arms, now the supporters of the arms of the "Imperial German Empire," are Barbarians, Salvage or Savage men, Sylvans, Orsons (or *Ur*sines, or "of the bears," therefore rough enough), men of the woods, or bovines, bulls, boasting the "horns,"—frequent in German heraldry, notably in the crests. The crest comes from *cresta, chrest i, cris:, chriss,* or "Christ." If the reader makes reference to the Imperial German crown he will again recognise the mythic "cleft," and also see its indications in the armorial ensign of the Austrian Empire, which is Oss*t-risch,* changed into Austerisch or *Aus*trian, and which possesses claims, indeed, to the Eastern, or the Byzantine Empire, which claims yet stand in dispute between the Emperor of Russia, the Emperor of Germany, and the Emperor of Austria. The King (not the Emperor, mark, for the Pope is the supreme "crowned one" in this dignified respect) of Rome —a title now non-existent—is properly the Cæsar, or the suzerain of the Roman Empire, the Holy Roman Empire; and as such the Emperor Napoleon the First, and also the Emperor Napoleon the Third (his uncle's imitator, or, as the French doubtless think now, his parody), sought to make each his son—the King of the Romans. The title of Prince of the Galles, or Walles, or Wales, and that of the Dolphin, or Dauphin, the title of the eldest son of the King of France, is similar to this.

P

the visionary mazes of the woven fabric of the writings of that sublime arch-mystic, Jacob Behmen, to whom, if he desires farther light and higher light, we refer the studious and inquisitive reader. None other than a studious (who must, therefore, be an inquisitive) reader ought to deal with these subjects, abstract and transcendental, and of course elevated and scriptural, and therefore undoubtedly Christian (though, in the philosophical sense, Christian) as they are. Here, in these histories, or in these accepted accounts of Saint Michael, the Archangel, and, in his impersonated soldierly shadow, or "double," conquering the Dragon in Egypt, and in his slaughtering of the Dragon, saving the Princess Sabra, or Seba, or Sheba (some examiners of the myths call her the "Queen Sheba," or Theba, or Teba, or the "Ark," epitomised or impersonated, in the feminine form—even King Solomon's "Queen of Sheba")—this Saint Michael and this Saint George may be safely allotted, also, to, and assigned important places in, the religious mysteries (certainly the Christian religious mysteries), gathered around, and constituting the meanings of the Holy Graël. The Holy Graël is the parent and producer of, and in its development grows into, and becomes the same thing as the "Round Table" of King Arthur, the British king. The Round Table was the consulting, astronomical, and astrological (clearly magic) disc, endowed with supernatural gifts, gained from Heaven through the prayers and the ministration of the enchanters, or sages, or magi. The Round Table was also a spiritual planetarium, a mirror emblematic of the whole circle of the terrestrial and angelic rounds, or circuits, or courses, or dominions of the "seen" and the "unseen" universe,—both the body

and the spirit of all that is, and the depository of all
prophecy, and of all magic, or the power of moving
Nature, or compelling Nature (under the will of God),
up to the exhaustion of this world's business, and the
passing up to the final consummation. Round this magic
table, or this stupendous round table, King Arthur and
his knights (each a champion and a saint, in the double
character derived from earth and from heaven,) sat, at
certain periods, to consult in solemn conclave, holding thus
a sort of inexpressible sacrament, "breaking bread" and
"drinking wine," and rendering the solemnity a sort of imitation "Holy Supper." This was imitated afterwards, in
all devotion and holiness, by that magnificent monarch of
England, King Edward the Third, who took the Round
Table as his model, and the knights of King Arthur's
court for the originals of his knight-companions, and
restored and amplified the "Round Table" in the "Most
Noble Order of the Garter," being himself the first
president and sovereign of it, elevating his son, the Prince
of Wales, to be the next to himself, and in the humblest
imitation of the divine gradations of majesty, seating his
"first-born" at the "right hand" of his father, and
gathering around him as peers, or as sages, champions,
angels, and saints, his chosen sacred "twenty-four,"
double the number of the apostles, and double the
number of the patriarchs or "children of Israel," because
this "twenty-four," or this number of twelve repeated
twice over, was supposed to be endowed with power in
a double capacity, and to stand representative of the night
and the day, or of the dark and the light (magic), sides
of a "true day," which, of course, consists of twenty-
four hours. In the last place, raising to the highest this

theory of greatness and power, Edward III. dedicates the
entire Order, with all its rites, _forms, sentiments, and
meanings, consecrating the whole, to the Virgin Mary as
the Patroness of the Sacred Order of the Garter,
"Keeper," or "Garder," she being the Queen of Heaven
and the Immaculate Mother of Jesus Christ, "Lord" and
"Saviour" before whom "every knee shall bow." Included in this universal obeisance are the rebellious
inhabitants—now mastered by Saint Michael—imprisoned
in the vast abysses of the nethermost "Hold"—namely,
Darkness and Matter—which is yet, transcendentally, the
rearmost side of Light. Light and Darkness are identical
in themselves, being only divisible in the human mind;
for, as the sophists contend, Darkness is but the reversed
side of Light, and, according to Robert Fludd, Darkness
adopted illumination in order to make itself visible.
Light, as the scientific philosophers know very well, is
material enough, although we lack such exquisitely
delicate balances as would be required to weigh it.

Both Saint Michael and Saint George are types. They
are sainted personages, or dignified heroes, or powers
apotheosised. They are each represented with their
appropriate faculties and attributes. These are reproduced
and stand multiplied—distinguished by different names—
in all the mythologies. But the idea regarding each is a
general one. This idea and representative notion is that
of the all-powerful champion—childlike in his "virgin
innocence"—so powerful that this God-filled innocence
(the Seraphim "know most," the Cherubim "love most")
can shatter the world (articulated—so to use the word—
in the magic of Lucifer, but condemned), in opposition to
the artful constructions, won out of the permission of the

Supreme—artful constructions ("this side life")—of the magnificent apostate, the mighty rebel, but yet, at the same time, the "Light-bringer," the Lucifer—the "Morning Star," the "Son of the Morning"—the very highest title "out of heaven," for in heaven it cannot be, but out of heaven it is everything. In an apparently incredible side of his character—for let the reader carefully remark that qualities are of no sex—this Archangel Saint Michael is the invincible sexless, celestial "Energy"—to dignify him by his grand characteristic—the invincible "Virgin-Combatant" clothed—(and yet suddenly interposes a stupendous mystery, a mystery which lies at the very root of true Buddhism and Gnosticism, for both, in their radical metaphysical bases, are the same)—clothed, and at the same time armed, in the denying mail of the Gnostic "refusal to create."* This is another myth, a "myth within myths," at the same time that it is a stupendous "mystery of mysteries," because it is so impossible and contradictory. Unexplainable as the Apocalypse. Unrevealable as the "Revelation."

The writings of Jacob Behmen abound with these strange contradictory theosophic speculations. This is truly the mysticism of the Gnostics, the Manichees, and Buddhists. It is also, in certain of its phases, the mysticism of the Platonists. It is precisely the reverse of those doctrines usually attributed among the learned to the Buddhists and to the reasoning philosophers among the professors of the forms of belief enumerated above. Facts may be right in philosophy, and yet the interpretation of some of the facts, or of most of them, may be

* The metaphysical foundations of Buddhism and Gnosticism are the same.

all wrong, because the inquirer's means of examination may be incommensurate or faulty in some principal respects, which may spoil all his deductions and conclusions, even in the instance of, otherwise, very clever men. Ambition and self-occupation and self-conceit are great deterrents in these respects. Even absolute ignorance has a great deal to do with such mistakes. For academic distinctions, in themselves, are not worth much.

But to resume with our ultra-metaphysical distinctions in the region of this (save for that leading mystic, Jacob Behmen, and for one or two others of a similar profoundly thoughtful character) unknown, and hitherto very superficially explored, "mystic anatomy." Women may be said to be "Men-Forward." Men may be said to be "Women-Backward." To comprehend all this it is absolutely necessary to possess an intimate acquaintance with the details of human anatomy, particularly in its most extraordinary and evasive forms. At the same time, nothing can be made of this reluctant and mysterious subject except by those gifted with powers of the keenest acuteness of observation and the most cautious judgment. Man and Woman are the same, in reverse of each other. The junction is the "shock." It is not seen, except by the mystic anatomists, that in the umbilicus and its extension instant and contemporaneous man, and every man, is (and must be) in continuous and corporeal direct descent from the prototype, and must consecutively, in an eternal chain of a line, until interrupted, propagate as a single being forward, while man is man, and the strange foreign race—to speak thus of man as an abstraction, from an altogether different standpoint from that usual—this strange foreign race, out of Nature, designated as Man, projected from the outside of Nature, as it were—*ab extra* of everything—like a human meteorolite (to put the case poetically) out of " unknown other worlds." Soul is nothing, body everything, in "This World." Body nothing, soul everything, " Out of This World." Woman (in pregnancy) is in a "magical" and, in one sense, unnatural state. This is, of course, apart from her being the means of perpetuating the race, which would almost seem the only object, as vouched in her peculiarities and by her personal configuration, of her being introduced into the world at all. It is certainly not for the pleasure of man, except in his state of mistake and of degradation.* A woman, about to give birth to a child, has ceased to be a real woman—in the exalted and intensifying sense—because she is not a woman properly— that is, a virgin. For a true, perfect woman—as a thoroughly independent entity—must be a virgin, because she has nothing to do with the opposite sex, having never been conjoined with the opposite sex, and having thus lost her perfectly independent singleness. A woman that is not a virgin is a spoiled woman. She is thus, in the admission or the supposition of all the peoples—highly so, in the ideas of all the most imaginative and refined nations. Woman forfeits her supernatural privileges and powers when she is despoiled—this in certain senses—of her virginity. She is said to be capable of clairvoyance— of prophecy—of divination—of supernatural insight;— said to be sacred and holy—to have powers over the spirits—in her condition of unconsciousness, or of maid-

---

* This is in the abstracted sense, of course, for we have elsewhere spoken of this pleasure as the very highest pleasure for man.

hood. These are great, wondrous endowments.* She
inspires all Nature with the fear of her. The poets have

* The prescription to King David, the "favourite of Heaven," be it
remembered, by his most skilful physicians, when the King was "old
and stricken in years," was the attendance and ministration of a maid.

" 1. Now King David was old, and stricken in years, and they
covered him with clothes, but he gat no heat. 2. Wherefore his
servants said unto him, ' Let there be sought for my Lord the King a
young virgin, and let her stand before the King, and let her cherish
him, and let her lie in thy bosom, that my Lord the King may get
heat.' 3. So they sought for a fair damsel throughout all the coasts
of Israel, and found Abishag, a Shunammite, and brought her to the
King. 4. And the damsel was very fair, and cherished the King, and
ministered to him; but the King *knew her not.*"—1 *Kings,* i. 1—4.

" Our author has given Abishag, the very fair damsel's adumbration,
most curiously.

" This danger of incontinence, King David being a very old man, is
another convincing argument that our author's cataplasm and remedy
and relief for the infirmities of old age is a virgin. For virgins are the
greatest temptations, very naturally, to the fault of incontinence.

" Now if the Sin of eating the fruit of the 'Tree of Knowledge of Good
and Evil' were the Scriptural Knowledge of a Woman (as is the opinion of
some learned men), a spotless Virginity may likely be the very thing in pro-
tracting that Evil Day of Man, which the beguiling of Woman by the Devil,
and her seduction by the Evil One, first brought upon the unhappy Man.

" Or admit, if our First Parents had not eat the 'Apple' (as most
Divines allow they really did), Man might have been conceived without
sin, and Woman might have brought forth without sorrow; this and all
other Acts being naturally performed, according to the Will of his
Creator, as the Sun goes round without sin, but that, by the Fall, Will
and Pleasure, and particularly this form of delight, has become sinful
and atrocious; and Lust has grown exorbitant and dominating over
everything in the world. When perhaps this natural instinct—before
the 'Fall'—was a pure, innocent, natural propensity, as for the Stars to
keep their courses. Even in Nature, every way corrupted by these
means, the Remedy is highly rational. For, in this case, the Virgin
heat and uncontrollable desires, irritated and exalted by the juxtaposition and contact of Man, however thus old and physically incapable,
exerts itself magnetically and sympathetically, spurred by the abounding

feigned that a naked woman, if a maid, can walk through the world, and that all Nature will thrill and tremble at

fancies of inventive and imaginative Woman, luxuriating in the feeble object thus only accidentally, grudgingly, and enviously afforded, exerts itself by its magic invisible expansion, radiation, and incubation (woman becoming the ' man' in force here, let it be carefully remarked) ; and then she so acts, with that vigour sent forth outwardly in her instinct of delight (contrived by Nature), in seeking to reproduce and to multiply, notwithstanding the useless, old, expended form presented to her, so that her own excitement at disappointment reinforces her power by implying to it the air of fury. Now the remedy and the restoration to health and strength of the aged Man in this vivifying, singular adminis- tration of the matchless physician (woman), who prescribes the remedy, is found in the fact that the Virgin expands that vigour outwardly, in her instinct mechanical (the gift of cunning Nature) for preserving her decaying species, her ' longing,' as it is called, which springs from her intense desire to produce of herself, and to give her likeness to the world. Here springs all the end of humanity. Thus the woman's powers and incitements find their escape and safety outwardly, which she would otherwise consume and use up, according to her nature, inwardly in procreation, the natural intention of her by her Divine Author. And on the other, this ' Old Dust and Ashes,' this ' Old Man,' this ancient ' stump with not a green leaf upon it,' may, by his concubine, full of spirits and vitality, have sparks of reanimation kindled in him (a new *elixir vitæ*), so as to keep the embers alive, that, for want of the fuel of life, are not able to break out into the grand magical flame of Lust, however eager and willing in intention, although insufficient to take green wood or powder (the wrong sort of powder) of wood. But if the Old Man's Vital Flame, thus trembling and lambent, flickering, so to say, over himself, should proceed to try to animate posterity in over-stimulus—tempted to destruction by the Devil—he must only expect his own speedy Extinction, and instead of re-acquiring new life, he must die outright. Thus the woman, however beautiful and tempt- ing, must be sacred to him, and (aided by the angels, who will help him in his refusal and continence) he will forswear her."—"*The Cure of Old Age and Preservation of Youth.* By that great Mathematician and Physician, Roger Bacon. Edited by Richard Browne, M.L. Coll. Med. Lond. London, Printed by Thomas Flesher, St. Paul's Churchyard, 1683."

her, and bow before her and worship her; that the devils
will fly from her face, and the wild animals crouch at her
feet; the angry thunders of Heaven be stilled, and the
bright sun—and, still more, the moon, because the moon
is the genius, and (mysteriously and mythically) the
maker of woman—beam forth.

> " 'Tis said that the lion will turn and flee
> From a maid in the pride of her purity."

And yet—to set against this—perpetual maidhood, or
even prolonged maidhood, is impossible to woman, except
as attended with unutterable mischiefs, amongst which, as
certainly not the least, will be reckoned, even in the best
regulated female mind, that of the almost certain ruin
of her beauty. These facts and theories—and more
facts and theories that lie behind and press upon one
in their number—furnish problems and wonderings as to
what should really be, as Nature intended, or as con-
ducive to the general vital policy, or of the preternatural
intentions in regard of her; whether the lines of probability in regard to woman's life in the world—beautiful
and ruinously seductive as woman is to man—lead up
to distrust if she be, or to the conclusion that she is
not, intended for personal rigid holiness, for the putting
aside and denial, with the terrors, both to woman and
man, which correspond with this uncomfortable fixedness
of her fate; or whether the instinctive desires and prepossessions should be allowed (and enjoined), with full
scope accorded; and whether, in a new order of things,
free licence and absolute cosmopolitism should become
mode and manners, introducing to as equally great, or
worse, dangers and to spiritual demoralisation, with no
reference to any responsibility of man, and to his

absolute ruin in other ways. We hope no time like this will arrive—even in America, where there is most danger.

But to return, and, in a certain measure, to repeat. A woman that is not a virgin is a "spoiled woman." She is a "victim:"—hence (in visible forms) her investment in white from time immemorial at her bridal or betrothal; for white was the colour of the victims among the Greeks and Romans, even among the Christians. She is not man, of course, because man is by Nature barren, though, if the "First Woman" was achieved out of the body of "Man," as we are told in Scripture, the first man could not have been barren, but must have been capable, in some incomprehensible manner, of reproducing his own kind. Man must, therefore, originally have been fertile, even in this very important and extraordinary respect, at least in this first instance, and even in this especial exclusively feminine characteristic. We must accept this as the true reading of the story of the Garden of Eden, unless we construe these portentous particulars as allegory, conveyed in the terms, and by the means, only possible. The imagination of man is always baffled in his conception of a miracle. But the whole of this singular side of life, through whatever interpretation we may place upon it, or however we may seek to justify to ordinary reason even the natural phenomena wherewith we are all so familiar, which show has become so continual, and is so inseparable to us, that we pay it no attention, and never recur with a "side glance" to it ("wondering at the wonder," as we may say); the whole of this side of life, as we safely declare, is magical, therefore miracle: therefore, being miracle, certainly not

Nature, because it is unnatural, as common sense understands Nature.

In regard to Woman—all her peculiarities and sympathies, her weakness and her unworthiness, her magic inferior nature, and her magic sinister, and yet heavenly (as the assuasive to the inherent brutality of man) superior nature, arise out of this fact—of her being under man, of her being the subject and not the object of creation.

> "*Mrs. Quickly.* Say—what thing?—what thing?
> "*Falstaff.* What thing?—Why—
> "A 'Thing' to thank God on!"

This, as thus put forward, is a jeer of Shakespeare, but it contains profound philosophical truth as to the real character of woman, apart from her magic excellence, from the magical point of view,—apart from her sex altogether.

Again, the act of generation, the most resistless morsel in the Devil's "armoury of temptations," as it has ever been found in all ages all over the world, and which has seized to itself the highest idea of beauty which the mind and the eager sympathies of man have been ever able to achieve (blind, and mad, and a delusion as, in reality, it is), this first idea, in the earliest age, and grasp at the "unattainable," is, at the same time, man's last snatch, in age, at the ultimate departed joy (when power has gone, even in remembrance), and it is the last cling for felicity that flashes up out of vitality in the expiring embers of surrendering age! In the old days—in the ancient Pagan times—in the highest cultured, in the most poetic classic periods, this link between earth and heaven—as it may most truly be called—was sacred—was an act of worship, —it is so intimated in all the myths and mythologies. It was a sublime religious "rite" in the old classic times, as also among the Jews. The Jews were always a very lustful people. There are certain natural reasons which render this tendency peculiar and remarkable in them. It is very generally admitted that, also, the Mahometans, among all the tribes and races, are very prone to libidinous indulgence. The act was sacred, as a rite, to the gods, in the ancient times. It was always looked upon as a sacred rite among the Christians. These ideas are strictly valid—although never taken notice of—even in these latter times, supposed to be exceedingly chaste, and accepted as scrupulously religious—abounding, nevertheless, in a vast amount of hypocrisy, as they undoubtedly do. At least, this in all men's private judgments and convictions about these sensual matters.

According to the Mahommedans all a woman's form is " magical," while the man's form is mechanical. All the Orientals, as is well known, hold the idea of woman very lightly. The woman's body the Mahommedan covers up and hides (as if Nature was ashamed of it) in public, and always at those times when circumstance or necessity compels her appearing in public. But for his own private gratification the Oriental reduces woman's form to its earliest nakedness, therefore to its magic, therefore to its primitive provocation in the beauty of its magic symmetrical bareness, when no eyes see but his own, offering her body as the means of his most exquisite enjoyment. The reader will probably perceive by this how exquisitely fine and delicate the tastes of some of the most refined of the Orientals must be, and will at once further apprehend the causes and reasons—and realise the justification—for the extreme, implacable, and relentless jealousy of the Turks and those other stubbornly sensual peoples. This universal passion affects nations and countries—as we know it does individuals—very differently. But amongst the Orientals, where "love rage" is very often the greatest of "rages," the cool inquirer and the correctly comparing and weighing philosopher will soon perceive how the greatest of danger must the most speedily spring up there in regard to that point where all the passions of men concentrate the most forcibly into fierceness. Oriental man, at this wholly-disclosed naked beauty of woman, when permitted to concentre all his uninterrupted, ravished attention on it, without distraction from outside things, is wholly occupied in his gaze, which sight of the glorious object—being complete—intensifies his pleasure and intoxication. The man of the East treats his lust for this beauty,—for all these enjoyments are not forbidden to him; for his heaven is composed of houris, and these enjoyed under the most delicious of circumstances, with ever-springing renewal of power and pleasure,—the Oriental—let it be remarked—indulges his vagaries of idea in these luxurious respects—his whims and his fancies, notably in the display of the limbs of the women in his seraglios, either freely displayed or temptingly and artfully semi-invested,—either for temptation to, or in rest from, or in solicitation in the future for, the exercise of his desires—in diaphanous or opaque drawers or trousers in the Harems. The Moslem, in fact—to put the case very roughly, but very truly, and very beneficially, in the right interests of this very delicate but extremely important subject (especially considering the tendency—doubtless lax and irregular—of the present times)—the Oriental—to use a coarse image—" devours" women in this way—"eating of his own flesh"—committing continually the first sin, and the capital sin—perpetuating the first abomination, making his women, in appearance (we will do him the justice to imagine that he stops short here), like men, yet remaining women,—in truth, the acme of lust. A lust "bred out of hell," and all the more hideous and Satanic because hinting of the dark Eblis (or the "bright Lucifer") by presenting itself in the lures of the beauty, snatched at in its magic, out of the splendours of heaven. The Moslem does not stop at women in the gratifying of his lewd, not amorous, propensities, but he extends his lust to all fit forms, and all forms that may present to him, in the masquerade of this feminine class. We have seen something of these strange aberrations from nature in the history of those debased masters of the world—as they esteemed themselves—the ultra-luxurious Emperors of Rome, in the high-class devotees among the Chinese, even amidst the common people, in the classic times, amongst the early races, in by-corners and in certain directions in the old world, as well as in the new, both in old and new times. These Orientals, of this irregular class, this debased brood, have recourse to either sex, or to neither sex, or to both sexes (accepted) in one. His own form, to make the indign side of it mysterious in character, the Moslem invests in long, dignified, concealing, muffling robes. He covers as much as he can of woman's form in public, as people hide away jewels and valuables which they wish to keep all to themselves, in accordance with the selfish, grudging suggestions of his avaricious sensuality, insisting on keeping, in his tyrannical, austere jealousy, all her beauty to himself, purposely to overwhelm himself, at the right times

for his self-gratifying purposes, with fleshly seduction.
He strips her, as much as is possible to him, in private,
to give edge and point and spur to his domineering lust,
which will know no check from magnanimity or forbear-
ance, and is stimulated by resistance. He covers as much
as he can of his own form, in his morbid and yet
highly-sensitive pride and dark, personal reserve, except
for war, when, of course, he astutely clothes and arms
himself fitly. The Turks are perhaps the most formally
decent and proud, in all the dignified, serious walks of life,
of all peoples. Mahomet had supernatural genius and
princely pride. The Turk bowstrings his enemies, giving
them thus the masculine *accolade*, and according them
the dignity of the honourably condemned. He accords to
his male criminals the privileges due to them as men, and
inflicts execution, implied under the terms of respect,
under pronounced and distinct and accepted methods of
execution, or of removal out of this world. He confers
the observances of execution, such as the honour of be-
heading, or by the methods of getting rid of his victim,
or the "devoted to death," put in practice by the Thugs,
who made a consecrative rite or sacrifice of the strang-
ling of their victims, or were even supposed to assist them
religiously in freeing them from the "animal rings and
purgatories," hindering them in their forward progress of
exaltation out of the condemnation which to these speculative Asiatics this earthly life meant. This sort of
honourable method of putting to death is practised in
the instance of males. But in the instance of females,
in the inspiration of the disdain of them, in Eastern
countries, the woman is removed out of the world as
not properly of it, and is therefore submitted to indign

methods of putting to death, if criminal,—such as are applied to the lower orders of creatures—not that the cruelty is greater, but that the carelessness and disregard are greater and more contemptuous.

The bowstring, or hanging, or execution by the sword or axe or poison, are the means employed to execute justice upon males among the Turks. There is consideration and a certain kind of honour in all these forms of death. Something of the same view of the inferiority of woman generally prevailed amongst the Romans, even in their most highly civilised times, under the Emperors. Thus it was against the Roman law to put a virgin to death, because a virgin (while such) was sacred, and not to be exposed to this last penalty, which was a degradation in a certain occult sense—that is, as a desecration from the sacredness of the idea of virginity, which was a matter for the gods, and a characteristic of the gods.

Farther than this—in regard of our own country. By the old constitutional, unwritten law of England women condemned to death were never hanged (like the canine creatures, for instance), but burned, which was the nobler penalty, applied to martyrs (to those who rebelled against the gods) and to those not guilty of any crimes of a low depth of enormity. Prior to this, execution by fire, and also to that, in many minds, the bitterer portion of the sentence, the previous outrage of them by the executioners, the first female Christian martyrs were subjected, many of whom are now reckoned among that glorious company of saints in heaven who laid down their lives in all the constancy of adhesion to their belief.

But the nobler and the more manly (that is, in the

sense worthy) punishments, the Turks inflict when their enemies are males, when they condemn their criminals. But another form of retribution is meted out to the women. Their last punishment and penalty varies. The master of his slaves must evolve fine distinctions out of the compassion of his own bosom, if he feels them. But he possesses the power to dispose of his property as he pleases; and, in the instances where he disdains, he destroys with cold-blooded indifference. He submits his delinquent women to the last punishment and penalty in his own contemptuous fashions. The Turk ties up his unfortunately lapsed women—women lapsed from the tyrannical bodily allegiance and serfdom to him, alone, in the relentless greediness of his inexorably selfish lusts—in the dark jealousy, and the slinking disdain of his own disappointed, particular desire to grasp all to himself—in the *sack*, and dismisses them into that—"outside of life," as we may, in our ignorance of it, in this, our real, genuine, sensible life, designate it :—whatever it be, in his carelessness of regard to it in the case of the female ; in respect of whom he will not even admit the idea of a soul :—thus he gets rid of the removed woman as a *thing*—as a thing to be delivered over into the void. Woman, in truth, owes her position in the social scale solely to the ideas of the Christians in these respects. Women owe everything to Christianity—both their honour and their place. And their allegiance and worship is due to the magnificent idea, occurring solely in the Christian gospel, of the immaculate birth of the Redeemer of Mankind through (of course, the "Virgin") Mary, the "Mother." It is a strange thing, that none of our acutest theologians (at all events, the modern

ones) will see—or, at least will not admit—that the
one half of the Christian Gnostic group are perfectly
right in assigning this assumed truth of the Miraculous
Birth of our Lord and Saviour, Jesus Christ, by the
Immaculate Virgin (incapable of sin, in this capacity) into
this "metaphysical show" of the world (as the Buddhists
contend that it is), in the only manner (that is, as the
super-excellent, first and best of Men) that can be entertained at all. God's knowledge is not man's "ignorance."
Where would the world have been, and where should
we men have been, had this been so? Except through
hopes, springing solely from and arising from the mysteries connected with the Virgin Mother—woman is a
lost creature. Western women—that is, Christian
women—rest thereon their hopes, and the excelling
dignity (more than that of men, according to Cornelius Agrippa) which the world ascribes to them, more
especially the privileges and advantages of marriage,
which, denying to them a succession of a partnership of
men—and of course the pleasures of boundless variety—
gives them *one* wherewith to grow old, and wherewith,
in their own indispensable interests, to be content ;—all
women of the Christian persuasion owe their position to
this elevation of the idea of "woman" in the person of
the Virgin Mary—first and holiest of her sex, in the
inexpressible greatness of her magic state. We advance
but a few steps in the examination of religious matters
before coming up, face to face, with a mystery—which
is soon found—before our eyes, and against our common
sense (which, in these matters, is *nothing*)—to convert,
and to metamorphose, into a miracle. Not all the logic
of the schools—not all the elaborate wisdom of the

dialectics, nor of the talking, disputative philosophers or scientific men, can move against this CERTAINTY. And the irresistible moral is caution and self-doubt—wherein we feel disposed to accept everything and deny nothing. The idea of a realised God—apart from the exaltation of man's attributes and of the human form (we use the word 'human' advisedly—omitting the distinction of male and female), reflection assures us is utterly impossible. If we begin to think otherwise we fall into the trap set by the devil, and veer about, perceiving that God—if we begin with our definitions—may be anything or nothing.

We again distinctly assert, beyond fear of contradiction, that women owe their rescue, in men's ideas, entirely to the operation of the Christian ideas, and especially to the influence of chivalry in the old days. The persuasions of the Christians in regard to the true character of women, and their place in the scheme of things, are quite different to those of the Asiatics. The Christians base their views upon the impulses and the heroic notions, emphasising action, as seen in chivalry and knight-errantry, which are especially instincts of the Cross. It is very similarly the case with the Israelites. It was the bringing of the Virgin Mary and the " Magdalen" to the front that raised woman, that elevated her out of the degradations customary in the East, and out of the humiliating and contemptuous idea entertained of the sex by the Jews. There is no limit to the repugnance felt to the feminine idea generally among the Jewish people : the exception is to the heroines, who passed out of the disabilities of women into the splendours of championship proper to man, saving their nation in the devotion of their self-sacrifice—proving triumphant, such

as Judith, Jael, Deborah, and others similar to these,
who, in this respect, from the greatness of their achievements, became, as it were, sovereigns, for sovereigns are
of no sex, and in every instance may well be classed as
of the nobler sex, or as " good as men." At least, these
grand Hebrew heroines became of almost as much dignity
and repute as the Jewish champions to the Jews.

These sexual notions constitute the groundwork and
form the difference between the ideas among the Turks
and those prevailing among Christians in regard to women.
These fixed persuasions, derived from their religions, are
the source and reason of the contrary character of the treatment of women and the opposite views in regard of them,
by the people of the two religions, Mahometan and
Christian—indeed, by the professors of all the Asiatic
forms of belief. In respectful and in truly reverential
consideration of these sexual facts (continually becoming
occult) lies the foundation of all faiths and of all philosophies starting from the views of the *true* character of that
creature much puffed up in his civilisation, man; which
true character is, in reality, sufficiently low. We believe
that in the progress of the ages man has strayed away
from the original enlightenment, and that, ceasing to be
the heaven-seeing and heaven-receptive child, nearest to
the truth in the child's instincts, impressionable to heavenly
or angelic influences, man has become devil-endowed in
knowing; eating, as it were, the second Apple.

The whole magic, real side of human nature, and the
supernatural origin of that strange universal feeling, which,
from want of a better knowledge of what, in reality, it is,
we call *shame*, in regard to particular parts of our persons,
prove to the more profoundly thoughtful, and to those

who can abstract themselves from the usages of life sufficiently to take independent views, "from the outside," of their form and "make-up" (as it were), and wonder at the uses, and the disgrace, in the exercise of certain of their members—seized and adapted to answer extraordinary objects, having nothing to do with the person's individual well-being—all these strange matters startle and confuse, and supply the deepest problem in life.

The idea of the shame of the Act is the foundation of not only all celibacy or monasticism, both sacred and profane, and penance, or self-immolation—in other words, of "sacrifice"—but at once explains and justifies—even enjoins and orders it;—at all events, in all instances of special self-devotion to the service of God-Almighty—for Priests, and those to whom are committed the guardianship, and, at the same time, the *exercise* of the mysteries. For this reason, in the Romish Church, the cup of the "Sacrament," the Cup of the "Holy Spirit of God," or of the "Holy Ghost," is denied to the Laity—very properly and obviously. For this sacred, mystic reason—also very properly and obviously—the "Blessed Cup," the "*Sang Real*," or "Blood Royal" mystically in the elaborate and splendidly-magnificent "parade of solemnities" of the High Christian Church—however, not acknowledged, and considered an illegitimate, or bastard, daughter of the Established Church, or Parliamentary Protestant Church (an impossible Church)—contains "mixed potation," or "water," mixed with and diluting or tempering the "wine," the power, and the meaning of the full mystery conveyed in the Wine being *veiled*, even to the celebrants.

The Brothers of the "R. C." sought resolutely to

stand aloof from all mankind in these respects—of mastering their passions in regard to women. They laboured —and laboured successfully in their own way—to trample upon the base parts of their nature—to avert from the temptation and to refuse the embraces of women. The histories of all the saints supply abundant proof of this ; the foundations of the principle of monasticism rest, all over the world, on this abnegation.

Curiously enough, in the observances of all peoples, especially in the instance of the older peoples, and those of the most highly refined and cultivated disposition, this hermit-like life, though contrary to nature [even contrary to orders], was esteemed the holiest. There has always been a certain sort of apology offered to nature—as if nature were offended at, and only permitted in a certain coy and reluctant way, the kind of indecent thing ; as if nature were frowning and deprecating, assenting in one sense, and refusing in another ; disapproving, even denouncing. There has always been a sort of amiably apologetic idea about marriage. There has been implied (upwards) the plea, or the plaint of necessity :—certainly of necessity, but, just as certainly, of necessity seeking indulgence. Marriage, and the other tender relationship—so accentuated, but so signally snatched, and so transitory (happily so transitory, for otherwise it would make " short work" with man—and woman, too !—and would soon kill) ; these pleasures are begged for with downcast eyes, and with hesitation and shamefacedness, as a boon—as a boon indeed !—in regard of which, every fibre of man—and of woman, too—particularly of the youth of either sex—passionately clamours. To the body of man—and of woman also—that very fine work (the handiwork ?—

yes, doubtless, the handiwork !)—of Nature, this so very intimate halving or coincident magic junction, or fellowship " out of" nature, and " in" nature—and this at the " same time") is the only heaven—at all events, is the best heaven. The Bride has always been ashamed of herself. She has always needed consolation and simulated retrieval, as if to condone penalties. Some of the quaint forms of marriage, also, speak of the need of (and of the possible proffer of) instant rescue—even at the instance of, and as by the ordainment proceeding from, Nature herself, or from the authors of nature. However, from the strictly phallic, and from the Priapean view—which is an universal one—the Bride has elected (hence come the prodigious responsibilities of the man) to forego the rights of pleased exercise which her mother, Nature, has conferred upon her—rights extending to an infinitely wider privilege than those assigned to the one man chosen (and, perhaps, the man soon to prove traitorous to his undertakings—which may, perhaps, be beyond him). She, herself, has, perhaps, in her fond and foolish, over-hasty trust, and ignorant and inconsiderate self-abnegation resigned her rights to a community general in regard to husbands, or efficients equivalent. This will depend upon the view taken of the natural rights of women in regard to the very proper, and very natural, and incontestably inalienable privileges, of her claims, as a woman, on man.* All women—of course all the girls,

* Mr. Long's " Babylonian Marriage Market" (sold in 1882 to the Holloway Institution for 6,300 guineas) was absurdly named, seeing that the subject had nothing whatever to do with marriage. Probably the aristocratic and other crowds who filled the Royal Academy and gazed with curiosity upon this picture would have been shocked had it been described under its right name. When

and the young women—may be, in some senses, con-

will England—and educated England, in the greater degree—become less hypocritical and more candid ? The scene represented in the picture related to the historical, legalised indulgence of the merest accidental lust (an awful tyranny), in fulfilment of a sacred obligatory law in Babylonia. We only wonder whether the crowds of ladies, old and young—most diligent in the avail of glasses to realise particulars—these mostly fashionable ladies, who crowded round and admired this picture (which fell far short indeed of its object), were aware of its real meaning.

The following is the authentic account of this slavish (but in its intention sublime) solemnity, as practised by the Babylonians. It is strictly true in all the particulars as given by Herodotus.

"Les Babyloniens," says Dulaure, "ont une loi bien honteuse : toute femme, née dans le pays, est obligée, une fois dans sa vie, de se rendre au temple de Vénus, pour s'y livrer à un étranger. Plusieurs d'entr' elles, dédaignant de se voir confondues avec les autres, à cause de l'orgueil que leur inspirent leurs richesses, se font porter devant le temple dans des chars couverts. Là, elles se tiennent assises, ayant derrière elles un grand nombre de domestiques qui les ont accompagnées ; mais le plupart des autres s'assèyent dans la pièce de terre dépendante du temple de Vénus, avec une couronne de ficelle autour de la tête. Les unes arrivent, les autres se retirent. On voit en tout temps des allées séparées par des cordages tendus. Les étrangers se promènent dans ces allées, et choisissent les femmes qui leur plaisent le plus. Quand une femme a pris place en ce lieu, elle ne peut retourner chez elle que quelque étranger ne lui ait jeté de l'argent sur les genoux, et n'ait eu commerce avec elle hors du lieu sacré. Il faut que l'étranger, en lui jetant de l'argent, lui dise : 'J'invoque la déese Mylitta.' Or les Assyriens donnent à Vénus le nom de *Mylitta.* Quelque modique que soit la somme, il n'éprouvera point de refus : la loi le défend ; car cet argent devient sacré. Elle suit le premier qui lui jète de l'argent ; et il ne lui est permis de repousser personne. Enfin, quand elle s'est acquittée de ce quelle devait à la deese, en s'abandonnant à un étranger, elle retourne chez elle. Après cela, quelque somme qu'on lui donne, il n'est pas possible de la séduire. Celles qui ont en partage une taille élégante et de la beauté ne font pas un long séjour dans le temple ; mais les laides y restent davantage, parce qu'elles ne peuvent satisfaire à la loi. Il y en a même qui y demeurent trois ou quatre ans."—*Herodote, Clio,* chap. cxcix.

sidered as the universal children of ~~Venus~~—in this way ;
the great Mother, the grand, sublime Isis ; she whose
" veil"—in magic awe—is never to be removed—because, according to the mythologists, the consequences
would be only too fatal. Venus is the " flower of
heaven." This is the Venus-Pandemos ;—for the goddess, Venus, has many names. In truth, Venus, in some
of her phases, is double-sexed. There is the " Venus
barbata," or " <u>bearded Venus</u>," in the same double way,
and with the same double meaning, as, in the mythological sense, there is not only a Lu*na*, but a Lu*nus*. The
name Ven*us*, in itself, is masculine in its termination, and
the goddess becomes the god, and the god the goddess,
sometimes. The chief or leading Venus is, however, in
the most beautiful and glorious relationship to man—the
" Venus Victrix," the Venus-Pandemos—that is, the
patroness of all free women ; or, to sum up in one superlative word, Venus is the Grand " Hussey" of the World.
Now, in regard to the loftiest rights born with every
female, and the talismanic tokens of which she bears, and
parades (secretly) throughout the worlds, both visible
and invisible—both natural and supernatural, both human
and divine—she puts in evidence, in the establishment of
which she can appeal to her personal proofs—unless
(which happens, sometimes) she be defrauded by nature
as " spoilt work"—which marshalling of proofs (as we
repeat) is irresistible and triumphant in any court of the
world, and has always so been—in any court, and before
any judgment-seat, Human or Divine.

There is a large amount of hypocrisy in thus seeking
to deal, in the selfish, apologetic, bargaining way, about
the matters which are referred, coarsely, to the promptings

of the "flesh." In fact, they are simply promptings to
signal honour and glory, and delight—but this, let it be
remarked, in the natural sense. Now, the natural and
the supernatural are utterly opposed, except where they
stand as one, in magic and miracle—in regard to which,
it is contended, throughout our book—and as the text of
our book—that both are *real things.* We—that is, the
human race—as it were, protests to the superintending
Providence in regard to this desire of the body—found
so supreme a temptation that the assault of it will even,
in the instance of the most faithful man of God, endanger,
or rather shake heartily, even down to the wholly
" toppling down" thereof—his faith and his allegiance.
Awful thought ! We are prepared to swear a thousand
oaths that we only wish it " this once ;" and we pray, as
we pretend, for the withdrawal of the attention meanwhile,
and for the averting of the eyes of the Deity—whatever
this unknown Deity may seem, or show, or disclose, or
" vouchsafe," or be to us—even for a short moment ;
otherwise we feel that we cannot " command ourselves,"
and we shall, in that unfortunate case, lay all the blame
upon " nature," or upon the God himself. We, as it
were, put the case to the superintending Providence—we
call " Him," or " It"—" Nature," because it then becomes clearer to our senses, and is more reconcilable to
our infirmities, which seek kinship and repose *in* nature,
and *by* nature. We call all this " outside"—which,
distrust and fear about it disturb ; we seek to enter this
court of the Mighty Judge by side entrances, and to
essay the " private access," in order to slink from the
terrors, and to escape, in our fear and self-inclining, the
challenge of those " Awful Sentinels" which stand armed

on either side of the legitimate, and only properly-authorised, entrance to the Tribunal. We call all of this "Nature," being reluctant to acknowledge the vivid vitality of the "Personality" of the Ruling and Governing God. Therefore we manufacture to ourselves all sorts of apologies and protestations about these certain questionable incidents of "marriage" (as they seem in human fear), and so forth; as if to ask so many sanctions of the Church to make it holy, never being satisfied, or feeling quite easy, until blessing after blessing is sought over it—the trespass of the desire to live, and to enjoy, as then the only limit—to ask but once; and then to beg the privilege, in the interest of humanity, to the obtaining of a representative of ourselves and the continuing of man, securing the privilege, out of the mercy and forgiveness of Providence, for forming such libidinous wishes, sprung as weeds only, fit for the fire, out of the "devil-sown" mortal field, left as the legacy of the "Enemy of Mankind" for the fated inheritors of that fearful field, of and for the children of Adam to inherit—the heirs of the "Curse."

There is nothing in the lower and sensible world that is not produced and hath its image in the superior world. Since the form of the body, as well as the soul, is made after the image of the Heavenly Man, a figure of the forthcoming body which is to close the newly-descending soul is sent down from the celestial regions to hover over the couch of the husband and wife when they copulate, in order that the conception may be formed according to this model. We have before declared, in this chapter on the mystic anatomy, enlarged upon by Cornelius Agrippa, that the human "act," by which the power of perpetuation has been placed in the exercise by man, and has been elevated into the irresistible natural temptation, is rightly a solemnity, or magic endowment, or celebration to which all nature not assents simply, but concurs, as the master-key, however blindly or ignorantly, or brutally often practised. The Sohar, iii., 104, a, b, declares that "At connubial intercourse on earth, the Holy One (blessed be He!) sends a human form which bears the impress of the divine stamp. This form is present at intercourse, and, if we were permitted to see it, we should perceive over our heads an image resembling a human face. And it is in this image that we are formed. As long as this image is not sent by God, and does not descend and hover over our heads, there can be no conception; for it is written, "And God created man in his own image" (Gen. i. 27). This image receives us when we enter the world, it develops itself with us when we grow, and accompanies us when we depart this life, as it is written, "Surely man walked in an image."

The followers of this secret doctrine of the Kabbalah claim for it a pre-Adamite existence. It is also called the secret wisdom, because it was only handed down by tradition through the initiated, and its whole story is indicated in the Hebrew Scriptures by signs which are hidden and unintelligible to those who have not been instructed in its mysteries. All human countenances are divisible into the four primordial types of face which appeared at the mysterious chariot-throne in the vision of the prophet Ezekiel—viz., the face of man, of the lion, the ox, and the eagle. Our faces resemble these more or less according to the rank which our souls occupy in the intellectual or moral dominion; and physiognomy does not consist in the external lineaments, but in the features which are mysteriously drawn in us.

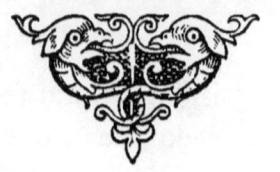

APPENDIX.

ONE day as Mahadeva (Siva) was rambling over the
earth, naked and with a large club in his hand, he chanced
to pass near the spot where several Munis were perform-
ing their devotions. Mahadeva laughed at them, insulted
them in the most provoking and indecent terms, and, lest
his expressions should not be forcible enough, he accompanied the whole with significant signs and gestures. The
offended Munis cursed him, and his Linga or Phallus fell
to the ground. Mahadeva in this state of mutilation
travelled over the world bewailing his misfortune. . . . .
The world being thus deprived of its vivifying principle,
generation and vegetation were at a stand Gods and
men were alarmed, but, having discovered the cause of it,
they all went in search of the sacred Linga, and at last
found it grown to an immense size and endowed with life
and motion. Having worshipped the sacred pledge, they
cut it with hatchets into one-and-thirty pieces, which,
polypus-like, soon became perfect Lingas. The Devatas
left one-and-twenty of them on earth, carried nine into
heaven, and removed one into the inferior regions for
the benefit of the inhabitants of the three worlds. . . . .
To the event related is ascribed the origin of the
Linga or Phallus and its worship. It is said to have
happened on the banks of the Cumud-rati or Euphrates,

and the first Phallus was erected on its banks (under
the name of BALESWARA LINGA). This is confirmed
by Diodorus Siculus, who says that Semiramis brought
an obelisk from the mountains of Armenia and erected
it in the most conspicuous part of Babylon. It was
150 feet high, and is reckoned by the same author
one of the seven wonders of the world. The Jews,
in their Talmud, allude to something of this kind;
speaking of the different kinds of earth of which the
body of Adam was formed, they say that the earth which
composed his generative parts was brought from Babylon.—(Wilford, *A Dissertation on Semiramis. Asiatic
Researches*, vol. iv., pp. 367—378.)

Henry O'Brien quotes from Sir William Jones an
account of attempts made against Sheevah (Siva) by a sect
of hypocritical devotees whose practices he had exposed.
It concludes as follows:—"Not yet disheartened by all
these disappointments they collected all their prayers,
their penances, their charities and other good works, the
most acceptable of all sacrifices, and, demanding in return
only vengeance against Sheevah, they sent a consuming
fire to destroy his genital parts. Sheevah, incensed at
this attempt, turned the fire with indignation against the
human race, and mankind would have soon been destroyed
had not Vishnou, alarmed at the danger, implored him to
suspend his wrath. At his entreaties Sheevah relented.
But it was ordained that in his temples those parts should
be worshipped which the false devotees had impiously
attempted to destroy." And accordingly the Eastern
votaries, suiting the action to the idea, and that their
vivid imagination might be still more enlivened by the
very form of the temple in which they addressed their

vows, actually constructed its architecture after the model of the *membrum virile*, which, obscenity apart, is the divinely-formed and indispensable medium selected by God himself for human propagation and sexual prolificacy. This was the Phallus of which we read in Lucian, in his treatise ' De Deâ Syriâ,' as existing in Syria of such extraordinary height, the counterpart of our Round Towers, and both prototypes of the two ' pillars' which Hiram wrought before the temple of Solomon." (O'Brien, *Round Towers of Ireland*, 100-101.)

A Frenchman recently returned from India, and who furnishes me with these details, assures me of his having furtively penetrated into the most secret sanctuary of the pagoda of Treviscare, consecrated to the worship of Siva, and having seen there a kind of granite pedestal consisting of a large base and a column supporting a basin, from the centre of which runs vertically a colossal Lingam about three feet high. Below, in the stone forming the base, is a large cleft representing the female sex. In this sanctuary, which is only lit from above, and on this stone, the priests of Siva initiate into the mysteries of love the young devidanis or dancing girls of the temple.— (Dulaure, *Histoire Abrégée de différens Cultes.*)

Unlike the abominable realities of Egypt and Greece, we see the phallic emblem in the Hindu Pantheon without offence, and know not, until the information be extorted, that we are contemplating a symbol whose prototype is indelicate. Obelisks and pillars, of whatever shape, are symbols of Siva or Mahadeva. He is Fire, the destroyer, the generator, and the conical or pyramidal shape being the natural form of fire, is applied to its representative and symbolised by a triangle apex upward. As the deity presiding over generation his type is the Linga, almost the only form under which he is reverenced. It is also, perhaps, the most ancient object of homage adopted in India subsequently to the ritual of the Vedas, which was chiefly, if not wholly, addressed to the elements, and particularly to fire. There can be no doubt that at the period of the Mahommedan invasion the worship of the Linga was common all over India. Twelve great Lingas, which were objects of especial veneration, were at that time standing at widely distant places, one being at Rameriseram in the extreme south. Of these several were destroyed by the early Mahommedan conquerors, the most notable being that at Somnath, in Guzerat, demolished by Mahmud of Ghizni, concerning which Mirkhond, a contemporary of that conqueror, writes as follows :—" The temple in which the idol of Somnath stood was of considerable extent both in length and breadth. The idol was of polished stone. Its height was about five cubits, and its thickness in proportion ; two cubits were below ground. Mahmud, having entered the temple, broke the stone Somnath with a heavy mace. Some of the fragments he ordered to be conveyed to Ghizni, and they were placed at the threshold of the great mosque." The story of the idol being hollow and having a number of jewels hidden within it is a modern European embellishment, for which no foundation is discoverable. The Hindus insist that the blackstone in the walls of the Caaba at *Mecca* is a Linga or Phallus of Mahadeva, and that it was placed in the wall, out of contempt, on the establishment of Islamism, but that the newly-converted pilgrims would not give up its worship, and that the ministers of the new religion were consequently forced to connive at it. At present the principal seats of the Linga worship are in the north-east and the south of India, parts furthest removed from the early Brahmanical settlements, a circumstance serving to confirm the theory that this worship is a remnant of the ante-Brahmanical religion. The temples dedicated to it are square buildings, the roofs of which are round and tapering to a point. In many parts of Hindustan, and notably along the banks of the Ganges, they are more numerous than those dedicated to the worship of any other of the Hindu idols. Each of the temples in Bengal consists of a single chamber of a square form, surmounted by a pyramidal centre; the area of each is very small. The Linga, of black and white marble, occupies the centre; the offerings are presented at the threshold. Benares is the peculiar seat of this form of worship, the principal deity there, Visweswara, "the Lord of All," being a Linga, and most of the chief objects of pilgrimage being similar objects of stone. Some of these emblems, usually of basalt, are of enormous size, one at Benares requiring six men to encircle it. Lingas of the sort called *partha linga* are made for daily or temporary purposes by Brahmans or by women themselves, of earth or of the clay of the Ganges, and offered in Siva's temples, being thrown into the river after worship. The Linga is never carried in procession. Devi, Siva's consort, is often represented with a Linga on her head. One of the forms in which the Linga worship appears is that of the Lingayets, Lingawants or Jangamas, the essential characteristic of which is wearing the emblem on some part of the dress or person. The type is of small size, made of copper or silver, and is commonly worn suspended in a case round the neck, or sometimes tied in the turban. They are numerous in the Deccan, especially in Mysore, and also in Tehngana.—Moor, *Hindu Pantheon.* Coleman, *Mythology of the Hindus.* Wilson, *Sketch of the Religious Sects of the Hindus.* Wilford, *Dissertation on Semiramis,* &c.

The strictest chastity it prescribed to the priests of Siva, and when they exercise their ministry they are bound to abstain from all desires that the image they worship might suggest. As they are obliged to officiate in a state of nudity it follows that should they fail to control their thoughts, and should excited imagination transmit its influence to their external organs, the people, who could not fail at once to become cognizant of such prickings of the flesh, would stone them.—(Sonnerat, *Voyage aux Indes,* i., 311.)

PHYSIOLOGICAL CONTESTS—THE PELASGI—THE ROUND TOWERS OF IRELAND—ADORATION OF THE VULVA.

There is a legend in the Servasaru of which the figurative meaning is obvious. When Parvati (Devi) was united in marriage to Mahadeva (Siva), the divine pair had once a dispute on the comparative influence of the sexes in producing animated beings, and each resolved by mutual agreement to create a new race of men. The race produced by Mahadeva were very numerous, and devoted themselves exclusively to the worship of the male deity, but their intellects were dull, their bodies feeble, their limbs distorted, and their complexion of many different hues. Parvati had at the same time created a multitude of human beings who adored the female power only, and were all well-shaped, with sweet aspects and fine complexions. A furious contest ensued between the two nations, and the Lingajas were defeated in battle; but Mahadeva, enraged against the Yonijas, would have destroyed them with the fire of his eye, if Parvati had not interposed and appeased him; but he would spare them only on condition that they should instantly leave the country, with a promise to see it no more, and from the Yoni, which they adored as the sole cause of their existence, they were named Yavanas. . . . There is a sect of Hindus who, attempting to reconcile the two systems, tell us, in their allegorical style, that Parvati and Mahadeva found their concurrence essential to the perfection of their offspring, and that Vishnu, at the request of the goddess, effected a reconciliation between them; hence the navel of Vishnu, by which they mean the *os tincæ*, is worshipped as one and the same with the sacred Yoni.—Wilford, *On Egypt and the Nile. Asiatic Researches*, vol. iii., pp. 361—363.)

The modern Hindu phallic worship is mainly of this type. "The Argha, with the Linga of stone, is found all over India as an object of worship; it is strewed with flowers, and water is poured on the Linga. The rim represents the Yoni" (Wilford, *On the Sacred Isles in the West. Asiatic Researches*, vol. viii., p. 274). "The Linga, the immediate type of the regenerator Siva, is generally represented in mystical conjunction with the Yoni and Argha. . . . . If he dig a pond, the Hindu, if a Saiva, imagines it a type of the Yoni or Devi, and cannot fully enjoy the comfort it offers him until it be reunited to the other types of elemental nature. After numerous ceremonies, a mast is, on a lucky and sacred day, inserted into the centre of the mysterious Yoni or tank. The mast represents the Linga or Siva, and now the typical reunion of the original powers of nature is complete. The last ceremony of placing the Linga or mast is commonly called the marriage of the Linga and Yoni. Strictly speaking, the brim of the tank is the Yoni, its area the Argha. In front of most temples of eminence is seen a tank, some of them exceedingly beautiful, and in the centre of the tank a mast, generally with wooden steps nailed up its sides, to facilitate ascent to its cross-trees, for the purpose of hoisting a flag or decorating the Linga or mast with garlands of flowers, or sprinkling it with water, or placing lights on it. In some temples Devi is exclusively worshipped by her votaries, the Sactis, and the tanks attached to such temples have no mast or Linga."—(Moor, *Hindu Pantheon*, 385—390.)

The Phallic, and at the same time Persian, origin of those remarkable monuments, the Irish Round Towers, has been most exhaustively demonstrated by Henry O'Brien. According to him they were erected by a colony of the Tuath-de-Danaans, or *Lingam*-God-Almoners, who, fleeing from Iran, the ancient name of Persia, in consequence of the victories achieved by their rivals, the Pish-de-Danaans, or *Yoni*-God-Almoners, settled in Ireland. The names Fiadh-Nemeadh, or Fidh-Ne-mead, given to them in early Irish annals, he translates as Consecrated Lingams, Fidh being the plural of Budh, which signifies not only the sun as the source of generation, but also the male organ. He continues :—" The Round Towers of Ireland were specifically constructed for the twofold purpose of worshipping the Sun and Moon —as the authors of generation and vegetative heat—and from the nearer converse which their elevation afforded of studying the revolutions and properties of the planetary orbs. . . . . Having been all erected in honour of the Budh or Linga, they all partook of the phallic form; but as several enthusiasts personified this abstract, which, in consequence of the mysteries involved in the thought and the impenetrable veil which shrouded it from the vulgar, became synonymous with wisdom or wise man, it was necessary, of course, that the Towers constructed in honour of each should portray the distinctive attributes of the individuals specified. Hence the difference of apertures towards the præputial apex, the crucifixions over the doors, and the absence or presence of internal compartments. Those venerable piles vary in their elevation from fifty to one hundred and fifty feet. At some distance from the summit there springs out a sort of covering, which, accompanied as it sometimes is with a cornice, richly sculptured in foliage, in imitation *præputii humani*, terminates above in a sort of sugar-loaf crown. Their diameter at the base is generally about fourteen feet through, that inside measuring about eight, which decreases gradually but imperceptibly to the top, where it may be considered as about six feet in the interior. The distance of the door from the level of the ground varies from four to twenty-four feet. The higher the door, the more irrefragable is the evidence of the appropriation of the structure. The object was twofold: at once to keep off profane curiosity and allow the votaries the undisturbed exercise of their devotions, and to save the relics deposited underneath from the irreverent gaze of the casual itinerant. In their masonic construction there is nothing in the Irish Towers appertaining to any of the four orders of architecture prescribed by the moderns.

Prepared stone is the material of which they are generally composed, and evidently, in some instances, brought from afar. Sometimes also they appear constructed of an artificial substance, resembling a reddish brick, squared, and corresponding to the composition of the Round Towers of Mazunderan. With three exceptions all have a row of apertures towards the top, just under the pro-jecting roof. In general the number is four, and then they correspond to the cardinal points. In three instances there is one aperture towards the summit, in one instance there occur five, in one six, in one seven, in one eight apertures. Inside they are perfectly empty from the door upwards, but most of them are divided, either by rests or projecting stones, into lofts or stories, varying in number from three to eight. A striking perfection observable in their construction is the inimitable perpendicular invari-ably maintained." (O'Brien, *Round Towers of Ireland*, 61, 511—515.)

"When once the idea obtained that our world was female, it was easy to induce the faithful to believe that natural chasms were typical of that part which charac-terises woman. As at birth the new being emerges from the mother, so it was supposed that emergence from a terrestrial cleft was equivalent to a new birth. In direct proportion to the resemblance between the sign and the thing signified, was the sacredness of the chink, and the amount of virtue which was imparted by passing through it. From natural chasms being considered holy the vene-ration for apertures in stones, as being equally symbolical, was a natural transition." (Inman, *Ancient Faiths em-bodied in Ancient Names*, i., 415.)

The most ancient oracle and place of worship at Delphos

was that of the earth in a cave which was called Delphi, an obsolete Greek word synonymous with Yoni in Sanscrit; for it is the opinion of devout Hindus that caves are symbols of the sacred Yoni. This opinion prevailed also in the West, for perforations and clefts in stones and rocks were called Cavim Diaboli by the first Christians, who always bestowed the appellation of devils on the deities of the heathen. Perforated stones are not uncommon in India, and devout people pass through them, when the opening will admit it, in order to be regenerated.—(Wilford, *On Mount Caucasus. Asiatic Researches*, vol. vi., p. 502.)

Those prophetic women of Etruria designated Sibyls were, says O'Brien, "named from the same cause, being priestesses of the serpent—*i.e.*, the Sabh or Yoni. . . . . Pythia is exactly synonymous with Sibyl, meaning the priestess who presided over the Pith, which, like Sabhus, means as well serpent as Yoni, and the oracle which she attended was called Delphi, from De, divine, and phith, Yoni—it being but a cave in the shape of that symbol, over the orifice of which the priestess used to take her seat upon a sacred tripod or the religiously-emblematic pyramid." Dr. Inman says that in some places it was positively believed that "oracles of a peculiarly sacred nature were uttered by or through the vulva—*i.e., la bocca inferiore* of sibyls, pythonesses, or statues, or through clefts in the earth, as at Delphi." So, according to Major-General Forlong, the image of gold set up by Nebuchadnezzar on the plain of Dura, in the province of Babylon, was nothing but a phallic obelisk, as is shown by its height being sixty cubits and its diameter but six.—(*Rivers of Life*, ii., 304.)

LINGAM GODS IN GREAT BRITAIN.

Of the worship of the lingam General Forlong writes:
—"The generality of our countrymen have no conception
of the overruling prevalence of this faith and of the
number of its lingam gods throughout our islands. We
have been hoodwinked by the unjustifiable term 'crosses'
applied to the ancient symbols, which were always in the
form of obelisks or columns, and erected on prominent
places, as on knolls or open woodland sites, at cross
roads and centres of marts or villages. These emblems
were usually on a platform, raised one to five or even
seven steps. The only plausible reason for calling these
objects 'crosses' is that, being the Terminus or pillar-god,
he is usually found where fields, paths or highways meet
or cross, and because the new faith, as it triumphed over
the old, laboured to adapt, remodel and rename the old
columns and pedestals, to suit the new ideas, and in its
ignorance lost sight of the old deity, both in the Lingam
and Cross. The Fire-god might still have his niches on
these shafts, but with Virgins and babies, having circles
or haloes round them, and in company with rayed suns,
roses, triangles and horse-shoe forms, sufficiently appropriate to please the most fantastic Yonik or Ionian
worshippers; whilst arrows, or spear-heads and daggers,
were transformed into *fleur-de-lis* charms, grateful to
the vision of every Lingam devotee. The mutilation
and transformation were probably thought complete when
the columns were surmounted by a cross in the old Tau
or circle forms; which, however, only rendered the whole
more replete with Sivaik symbolism. As education, or
rather power to follow preachers, was attained, these

'Bethels,' or 'Village Crosses,' had roofs erected over them, or the roof was sprung from a point about three-quarters up the shaft, and carried on pillars and buttresses; the base was in some cases cut away to give more room and shelter for gatherings. Elsewhere the lingam was thickened or wholly encased, and so veiled by the ornate architecture of the time, that none but an awakened or practised and educated eye could detect the old symbolism. . . . . There is no mistaking the consistent conclusion of Britton's researches that 'the original form of all market crosses was simply a stem like Chester, or a tall shaft on steps.' It suits precisely this Innis Mura of Ireland, the god of the Roman nympheum, and all the unadorned Lingams of the East, as distinguished from the Sri-Lingams, or Linga-in-Argha. It was natural for the new priest to resort to the old and sacred places of meeting, at the foot of the old god's pedestal, and in time to erect there a canopy or shelter for himself and congregation. . . . . The shires of Glocester, Wilts, and Somerset, still claim over two hundred ' crosses and remains of crosses,' erected not only as the centres round which towns grew, but on hill-tops, islands, headlands, by sacred wells and on dangerous defiles. That these objects were a power in the land—recognised faith-emblems—we see from the fierce and persistent manner in which so many earnest Christian sects warred against them and all their ephemeral substitutes, such as maypoles, holy trees, and real crosses. The iconoclasts knew, what others in later times forgot, that these were no modern symbols, but emblems of their great enemy, that powerful faith which had struck its roots deep and widely into every sensuous and emotional feeling of man's nature." (*Rivers of Life,* ii., 381—383.) The author proceeds to give a brief account of a number of so-called crosses, the phallic origin of which may be visibly recognised. To quote a few of these descriptions may be interesting. "Glendower shaft at Corwen, Merioneth, a blunted column with a Yoni or Omega form at head, and a 'curious dagger' or spear, the conventional phallic device." "The Bisley shaft, Glocestershire, is a perfect Lingam, or the glans of one, such as we see on Assyrian altar sculpturings, and it is said to be built over a sacred well." "Tottenham, or Tothamshire, is a covering to the old Toth or Linga, and is now a solid spire, rising straight from the ground, the favourite form throughout the Eastern world." "The Nevern shaft, Pembroke, would pass for a good Mahadeva in any part of India." "Cheddar shaft, on the Mendip Hills, and Chipping Column, North Glocestershire, are or were the most perfect Mahadevas possible, both as to column and pediment, being raised on three steps, like so many Eastern lingams." "Glastonbury shaft was clearly a lingam or glans, such as Assyrians worshipped, but much more tapered, and ending in a nude figure. Britton wrote that it had fallen with the building surrounding it—the Yoni or cell—into complete decay in his time." (*Ibid.*, ii., 385-6.)

O'Brien points out the Phallic origin of the may-pole. The garland traversed by the pole was typical of the Yoni, the pole of the Lingam.

"In Southern England two names occur in later days, which seem to have somewhat replaced Taut,—Idris the Giant, and Michael the Archangel. The latter has been worshipped as a god at various times, and in widely different countries, but usually in or near to waters, as in

Armorika, Apulia, and on the sacred islet cone of St. Michael, where Romans, as well as Phœnicians, seem to have thickly congregated; and upon his mount St. Michael had also a chair, the Celtish euphemism for ark or womb. . . . . There are four great archangels which the world has, at different times and under various forms, accepted as Maha Kâls or Great Sivas. The Michael or archangel of Jahveh corresponds to the Gabriel of Ala, and is a god of 'Tumbas,' caves or arks, wielding a rod or Tri-Sool. . . . . Without Mahakal the labourer laboureth in vain, the fig-tree cannot blossom, neither shall fruit be in the vines, the labour of the olive shall fail, and the fields shall yield no meat, the flock shall be cut off from the fold, and there shall be no herd in the stalls. . . . . The Cornwall and Normandy mounts of St. Michael are comparatively close to each other, and the latter is also called a Mons Tumba. The faith ideas of these St. Michaels are ever the same. . . . . At Penzance, on Midsummer-eve, which good Christians prefer to call the eve of St. John the Baptist, the young and old of both sexes assemble with lighted torches; three tar-barrels erected on tall poles in the market-place, on the pier and in other conspicuous spots, are then urged into a state of vivid combustion. No sooner are the torches burned out (there is evident significance here) than the inhabitants pour forth from the quay and its neighbourhood, form a long string, and run furiously through every street, vociferating 'An eye! an eye!' ('Ishtar! Ishtar!'), and at length suddenly stop, when the two last of the string (a mighty serpent), elevating their clasped hands, form an eye to this enormous needle (Siva), through which the thread of populace runs, and thus they continue to repeat the game till weariness dissolves the union."—(*Rivers of Life*, ii., 244-249, i., 456.)

" In the churchyard of the village of Rudstone, in the East Riding of Yorkshire, there stands fixed in the ground a single upright stone. It stands about four yards from the north-east corner of Rudstone Church, which is situated on a high hill. Its depth underground is equal to its height above—a fact which was ascertained by Sir William Strickland in the year 1776. All the four sides are a little convex, and the whole covered with moss. It is of a very hard kind of stone. It is twenty-four feet long above ground, and it is five feet ten broad and two feet thick. The weight of it has been computed at upwards of forty tons. The village probably took its name from the stone. The word Rud in Yorkshire means red. It is spelt Rudstan, and often Ruddestan. Immediately adjoining to the town of Boroughbridge, in the North Riding of Yorkshire, and within about a mile of the ancient capital of Britain, Iseur, may be seen three similar stones, almost equally large." (Godfrey Higgins, *Celtic Druids*, lxxiv.) Here is a perfect Linga, and the association with the word red is very significant, this colour being used in anointing such stones. Higgins himself elsewhere says, " Throughout all the world the first object of idolatry seems to have been a plain unwrought stone, placed in the ground as an emblem of the generative or procreative powers of Nature."—(*Celtic Druids*, 209.)

" No one who has studied phallic and solar worship in the East could," says the author of *Rivers of Life*, " make any mistake as to the purport of the shrine at Stonehenge; although I confess the many accounts of it I had read had not awakened my attention to the real facts, so misleading are many European writers on this, to them, unknown lore. Here stand upright stones, forming, as it were, a circular shaft within a perfect *argha*, or spoon-like inclosure, and there to the eastward the holy ' Pointer' in the Os Yoni, over whose apex the first ray of the rising god of the midsummer solstice shines right into the centre of the sacred circle. . . . . In May, 1874, I made some very careful drawings of the Stonehenge shrine, and in the ' Pointer' at once distinguished ' the ever-anointed one.' He faces towards the circle, and in spite of every allowance for the accidents of weather-wear, &c., no one who has at all looked into Sivaik lore will hesitate for a moment in pronouncing him a veritable Maha-Deva; the prepucial lines have worn stronger than they probably first were, so that decency forbids our drawing the object larger. . . . . Those persons who have studied such monoliths all over the world in the market crosses and Hermai at cross-roads in Scythic and Celtish lands, and in the shrines of Greek and Latin races, will have no hesitation in agreeing with me."—(*Rivers of Life*, vol. ii., p. 233.)

PHALLIC WORSHIP AMONG THE GAULS.

A curious survival of the Phallic worship thus inaugurated in France subsisted down to a comparatively recent period. The first Bishop of Lyons, Potin or Photin, was honoured in Provence, Languedoc and the Lyonnais, as St. Foutin. Under this name, the connexion of which with " foutre" is obviously the reason for his being thus selected, he replaced Priapus, whose attributes were conferred upon him, and whose outward semblance he usurped. To him was ascribed the power of rendering barren women fertile, of restoring exhausted manhood, and of curing secret diseases, and it was consequently the custom to offer to him, as to his predecessor Priapus, *ex voto* in wax, representing the weak or afflicted members. At Varages, in Provence, the floor of his chapel was covered with them, and when the wind happened to clash them together the thoughts of those paying their devotions to the saint were apt to be suggestively interrupted. At Embrun amongst the relics in the principal church was included the phallus of St. Foutin, and the worshippers of this, in imitation of pagan rites, offered libations to their idol by pouring wine on its extremity, which is described as being reddened by the practice. The wine was caught in a jar and allowed to turn sour, when, under the name of "holy vinegar," it was employed by women for a singular purpose. At Orange, in the church of St. Eutropius, was another phallus made of wood, covered with leather, and furnished with its natural appendages, which was highly venerated by the inhabitants of the town, but which was burnt by the Protestants in the market-place in 1562, when it emitted a very evil odour. At Puy en Velay barren women prayed to a St. Foutin, and scraped away an enormous phallic branch presented by the saint, believing that these scrapings infused in drink would render them fertile. Other Priapic statues were similarly converted into saints. At Bourg Dieu, near Bourges, the inhabitants continued to worship one existing, no doubt, from the time of the Romans. The monks not daring to put an end to such religious practices, converted it into St. Guerlichon, or Greluchon. Barren women flocked to the abbey to implore the saint's prolific aid and to celebrate a *novena* in his honour, and on

each of the nine days stretched themselves at full length
on his figure placed horizontally, and then scraped away
some particles from a part of his person as prominent as
the corresponding member in his prototype Priapus.
These particles in water constituted a miraculous beverage,
and the continued belief in their efficacy resulted in a
diminution of the member in question. At the commencement of the present century a statue of St. Greluchon
was to be seen, in the wall of a house at Bourges, with
its member almost entirely scraped away by female
devotees. St. Gilles in Brittany, St. Réné in Anjou,
St. Regnaud, and St. Arnaud, were similarly adored,
though in the case of the latter a mystic apron usually
shrouded the symbol of fecundity, and was only raised in
favour of sterile devotees ; its mere inspection was, however, sufficient, with faith, to effect miracles. Near Brest
stood the chapel of St. Guignolé, or Guingalais, evidently
derived from *gignere,* to beget. The phallic symbol of
this saint consisted of a long wooden peg traversing his
statue, and showing itself in front in a very salient fashion.
The local votaries scraped off the end of this miraculous
and never-failing peg, and these scrapings, mixed with
water, formed a powerful antidote to sterility, though
scandal credits the monks of the abbey with affording a
certain amount of aid in this matter. When by oft-
repeated scrapings the peg got worn away, a blow from
behind with a mallet brought it to its pristine prominence,
and thus another miracle was presented to the faithful,
whose devotion continued unabated till the middle of the
eighteenth century. Guignolet was also honoured at
Puy in the same way, the scrapings being infused in this
case in wine, and the *curé* taking care that the phallus was

always in a state of prominence befitting the saint's peculiar reputation, and although an archbishop in this instance tried to put a stop to the cult, it subsisted till the Revolution.— (Dulaure, *Histoire Abrégée de différens Cultes*, ii., 267, *seqq.*)

The enormous phallus of white marble found at Aix, in Provence, was an *ex-voto* offered to the deity presiding over the thermal waters, by a grateful or expectant patient. The bas-reliefs of the Pont du Gard and the amphitheatre at Nîmes show singular varieties of phalli, simple, double, and triple, with branches, pecked by birds, furnished with wings, claws, bells, &c. One is bridled and ridden by a woman holding the reins. At Châtelet, in Champagne, a triple phallus in bronze, with the central member in repose, and the other two in the fullest vigour, was discovered. One of the most singular monuments of this worship was found in an ancient tomb discovered near Amiens. It is in bronze, and represents a human figure in a walking attitude, half covered with the kind of hood called Bardocuculus. It is in two parts, and on removing the upper portion, consisting of the head, arms, and body, a Phallus hidden in its hollow is revealed, and appears standing on the two human legs. The chapter of the cathedral of Amiens preserved this in its treasury till the Revolution (Dulaure, ii., 240—245). Drinking-glasses made in the form of Phalli, such as were used in the mysteries of Colyth, have been discovered. In the museum at Portici, on the cover of an ancient vase, which seems to have been used for sacred purposes, is an enormous phallus, which a woman is embracing with her arms and legs; whilst another shows a dealer in phalli, offering a basketful of his wares to a woman, who exhibits evident delight at their extraordinary proportions.

PHALLIC IDOLATRY OF THE JEWS.

"No one can study their history, liberated from the blind which our Christian associations cast over us, without seeing that the Jews were probably the grossest worshippers amongst all those Ophi-Phallo-Solar devotees who then covered every land. These impure faiths seem to have been very strictly maintained up to Hezekiah's days, and by none more so than by dissolute Solomon. This king devoted his energies and some little wealth to rearing Phallic or Solo-Phallic and Fire shrines over all the high places around him, and especially in front of Jerusalem, and on and around the Mount of Olives. . . . . The builders of the shrines of the Tyrian Hercules were those whom this prince got in Hiram and his staff; and seeing Phallic and Sun-gods enshrined on all the mounts of 'the holy city,' Hiram would not forget, in constructing Solomon's temple, all the idolatrous forms of his own land. On each side of the entrance, under the great phallic spire which formed the portico, were placed two handsome phallic columns over fifty feet high, capped with lotuses encircled with pomegranates, a representation of the Queen of Heaven and of the gravid uterus, and the symbol of a happy and fruitful wedded life. . . . . The phallic columns were hung about with wreaths of chains, which always denote serpents. . . . . These columns were called, that on the right Jakin, or 'he that shall establish,' and that on the left Boaz, or 'in it is strength.' Syrian temples had two huge phallic columns in the vestibule, so that Jakin and Boaz in Solomon's shrine were strictly in keeping. The constant recurrence of two stones, whenever stones are required, is a strange but consistent idiosyncrasy of all phallic-worshipping races.

The temple was only 120 feet long, 40 broad, and 60 high, in two stories, while the porch was a large tower, 40 feet long, 20 broad, and 240 high! The Holy of Holies was cut off with golden chains from the rest of the inner temple, shrouded and bedecked with two hooded serpents, called Cherubim, and with serpent symbols. The carvings on the walls were symbolic palm-trees, open flowers and cherubim, &c. The temple was very like hundreds we see in the East, except that its walls were a little higher than usual and the phallic spire out of proportion. The Jewish porch is but the obelisk which the Egyptian placed beside his temple, the Boodhist pillars which stood all around their Dagobas, the pillars of Hercules, which stood near the Phœnician temple, and the spire which stands beside the Christian church. The little ark stands under the shadow of the great spire, and beside the real little ark within we have the idea repeated by the presence of Jakin and Boaz."—(Forlong, *Rivers of Life,* i., 213—219.)

HEBREW BAAL-PEGOR.

The ceremonies observed in the worship of Baal Phegor, or Baal Peor, have exercised the pens of several commentators. According to Philo worshippers presented all the outward orifices of the body. Rabbi Solomon Jarchi, in his Commentary on Numbers xxv., ascribes to them a still more indecent and disgusting practice. According to him the worshipper, presenting his bare posteriors to the altar, relieved his bowels, and offered the result to the idol, "Eo quod distendebant coram illo foramen podicis et stercus offerebant." Beyer concludes that the Moabitish women first prostituted themselves to the idol and then to the Israelites, and this view is held by St. Jerome, who, in his commentary on Hosea ix., represents the idol as having in its mouth the characteristic of Priapus, "Denique interpretatur Beel Phegor idolum tentiginis habens in ore, id est in summitate pellem, ut turpitudinem membri virili ostenderet." Inman, translating peor as "the opening of the maiden's hymen," and Baal Peor as "My Lord the opener," holds him to have been a Priapus, and adds: "From time immemorial the virginity of woman has been spoken of as her greatest treasure. Hence it has been claimed for the deity. In ancient times the claim was made by the god as personated by or inhabiting the body of his priest on earth. Sometimes the demand was made for the god as represented by his image, which was specially formed for the purpose."

HEBREW PHALLICISM.

Brugsch Bey, in his address regarding the Jewish Exodus, delivered at the Oriental Congress in 1874, said that "the serpent of brass called Kereh, or the polished, was regarded as the living symbol of God." A serpent and a pole for a perpetually recurring phallic emblem. It may generally be taken to represent the *membrum virile*, accompanied by the quickening or exciting passion. The Israelites had certainly no monopoly of it.

The exact shape and make of the image set up by Aaron to be worshipped in the wilderness has been greatly squabbled over by orthodox and unorthodox. The best Hebraists hold the translation 'calf' untenable, and even if it were probable that the Israelites, as has been alleged, had a recrudescence towards the faith of their loathed taskmasters the Egyptians, there remains the fact that the image of a calf holds no part in the mythological pantheon of these latter, whose adoration was paid to living bulls and cows. The most tenable view philologically is that something round or orbicular, possibly a cone like that symbolising Venus, is intended by the original word employed.

The ancient Jews had small Lares and Penates, or Yonis and Lingams. We have two instances of such in the idols of Rebeccah and the Queen Mother Maachah (1 Kings xv. 13)—that of the Queen is called a Miphlitzeth, or in the language of the Vulgate, a "Simulacrum Priapi." In those oscillations into idolatry, of which they were culpable from the very outset, they appear sometimes to have leaned to the masculine and sometimes to the feminine cult, though it may be said that generally the tribes preferred the worship of the female energies or of the Grove. The Ephod, like the Ark, is a feminine symbol, and Gideon's attack on the altar of Baal was an attempt to upset the worship of the Sun-god. Micah, having both Ephod and Teraphim, the latter being Lingams or penates, seems to have worshipped both organs. In latter times we find the dwellers on Mounts Moriah and Zion, Ebal and Gerizim, at constantly recurrent enmity, and different cults prevailing alternately or existing coevally. "Our inspection of and investigations regarding the sacred shrines in and about Jerusalem—and of many similar sacred hills in the East, where the votaries of the Right and Left Hand sects, Sivais and Vishnuvas, or Ion-im, have similarly determined upon a joint worship —has long convinced us that the Holy Sepulchre was the Lingam and Solar Fire shrine of the 'Secret God,' 'The Most High,' and 'Lord of all Holy Fires,' and that the great Omphik or Wombal Mount of *Muré* or Moriah was the Vishnuite shrine of Terra or Pârvatî, mother of all rounded mounts, especially those with caves and wells" (Forlong, *Rivers of Life*, ii., 583). The writer proceeds to point out very clearly the existing traces of such worship in either instance.

It is clearly established that the word "thigh," used in Genesis xxiv. 2 and xlvii. 29, is a euphemism for that member the præputial curtailment of which was a covenant between the children of Israel and the Almighty. The hand of 'the eldest servant of the house' and that of Joseph were placed respectively on the phallus of Abraham and of Jacob when the oaths referred to in the verses noted were taken. The practice still prevails. "When the Mamlouks appeared for the first time at Rahmanyah our pickets arrested a native of the district who was crossing the plain. The volunteers who took him asserted that they had seen him leave the enemies' lines, and treated him harshly, looking on him as a spy. Meeting them, I ordered him to be taken to headquarters. Reassured by the way in which he perceived I was speaking, he sought to prove that he was not a follower of the Mamlouks. Seeing that I could not understand him he lifted up his blue shirt, and taking his phallus in his hand, remained for a moment in the theatrical attitude of a god swearing by the Styx. His face seemed to say, 'After the terrible oath I am taking to prove my innocence, can you doubt it?' His action reminded me that in the times of Abraham the truth was sworn to by placing the hand on the organ of generation."—(*Mémoire sur l'Égypte*, part ii., p. 195.)

"There is a striking resemblance between the Hindoo

and the Hebrew myths. The first tells us that Maha-
deva was the primary being, and that from him arose the
Sacti. The second makes Adam the original and Eve
the product of his right side. After the creation the
Egyptian, Vedic, and Jewish stories all place the woman
beside a citron or pomegranate tree, or else one bearing
both fruits; near this is a cobra or asp, the emblem of
male desire, because these serpents can inflate and erect
themselves at will. The unopened flowers of the citron
and its fruit resemble a testicle in shape; the flower of
the pomegranate is shaped like a bell, which closely
resembles the female breast, and when arranged in
bunches of three, recalls to mind the phallic triad. The
fruit of the pomegranate typifies the full womb. The
eating of the apple is equivalent to receiving that which
is at this day, to many a young and fair daughter of Eve,
'the direful spring of woes unnumbered.' "—(Inman,
Ancient Faiths embodied in Ancient Names, i., 498-9.)

GNOSTIC RITES.

The belief and practices of some of the Gnostic sects
were most revolting. "The soul, according to the
Ophites, on its departure from the body, has to pass
through the regions of the Seven Powers, which it cannot
do unless fully impregnated with knowledge (gnosis),
otherwise it is seized and swallowed by the dragon-
formed ruler of the world (Satan Ophiomorphos), and
voided through his tail back upon earth, where it animates
a swine or other brute, and repeats its career once more.
But if filled with knowledge it escapes the Seven Powers,
tramples upon the head of Sabaoth, and ascends to the
eighth heaven, the abode of Barbelo, the Universal

Mother. But if convicted of having left any offspring upon earth, it is detained below until it has collected all of them and attracted them within itself. This 'collection of itself' was obtained by the observance of perpetual chastity, or rather (by the usual compensation) of all the unnatural vices that invariably spring from such an article of faith. If, however, a female of the congregation should allow herself to become pregnant, the elders caused abortion, and taking the fœtus pounded it in a mortar, together with honey, pepper, and other spices and perfumes. Then this 'congregation of swine and dogs' assembled, and each dipping his finger into the mess, tasted of it. This they termed the Perfect Passion, saying, 'We have not been deceived by the Ruler of Concupiscence, but we have gathered up again the backsliding of our brother.' .... In illustration of the punishment for leaving offspring behind, and so doing the work of the Demiurgus, they told a wild legend that Elias himself had been rejected from the gates of Heaven, though to his own conscience a pure virgin, because a female demon had gathered up his seed and formed infants therewith, which to his confusion she there produced in testimony. Hence the origin of the Succubæ in later times, although they were supposed to do the work of their father the devil in a different way, connected with his supposed relations to the witches whose lover he was *ex officio.*"—(King, *The Gnostics and their Remains,* 128.)

"The Nezaires or Nazarains form a special sect in Syria, and live scattered amongst Mahometans, Druses, and Christians. They adore God and believe in Jesus Christ as a prophet chosen to instruct mankind and give them law. They pray indifferently to the apostles, the Virgin, and the ancient prophets. They practise baptism by immersion, celebrate the Nativity, the Ascension, and some other of the festivals instituted amongst us. They have a singular one which they call by the name of the Womb. In this solemnity they salute women with a holy respect, and affectionately embrace their knees, whence comes their title Worshippers or Adorers of the Womb. Libertinage is elevated into a maxim by the Nezaires. Amongst other depravities they allow a plurality of wives. The day of the Circumcision, when their year commences, all the women are gathered together in the hall of sacrifice, the windows are closed, and the lights put out. The men then enter, and each takes by chance the first woman who comes to hand. This abomination is renewed several times during the year, and particularly at the festival of the Womb, in memory of the creation of man and woman. It is customary for the chief of the law to take part in it with his wife, obliged like any other woman to mingle with the crowd."— (Mariti, *Voyage*, vol. ii., p. 62.)

SYMBOL WORSHIP.

We come now to speak of what we may designate female emblems. It may easily be understood that few people, if any, would be so gross as to use in religious worship true simulacra of those parts which their owners think it shameful to speak of and a punishment or reproach publicly to show. . . . . "As a scholar," says Dr. Inman, "I had learned that the Greek letter DELTA is expressive of the female organ, both in shape and idea. The selection of name and symbol was judicious, for the word Daleth and Delta signify the door of a house and the outlet of a river, while the figure reversed represents the fringe with which the human Delta is overshadowed .... and typifies what is known to anatomists as the Mons Veneris, or the door through which all come into the world."—(*Ancient Faiths embodied in Ancient Names,* i., 158, 107, 146.)

"The female organs of generation were revered as symbols of the generative powers of Nature or matter, as the male were of the generative power of God. They are usually represented emblematically by the SHELL, or *Concha Veneris,* which was therefore worn by devout persons of antiquity, as it still continues to be by pilgrims and many of the common women of Italy. The union of both was expressed by the HAND .... which, being a less explicit symbol, has escaped the attention of the reformers, and is still worn as well as the shell by the women of Italy, though without being understood. It represented the act of generation, which was considered as a solemn sacrament in honour of the Creator."— (R. P. Knight, *On the Worship of Priapus,* 28.)

"The TRIANGLE, in the Old World, was a sacred form, representing the properties—capacity and dilatation—of the female symbol. When we speak of the symbolical marks of the Hindus we shall find the triangle, with the apex downwards, to be the appropriate symbol of Vishnu considered as the principle of humidity. To descend is the property of water, and it naturally assumes that figure. Nor is the triangle with the apex pointing upwards a less appropriate symbol of Siva as fire, it being the unvaried form of the igneous element, whose property is ascension."—(Moor, *Hindu Pantheon,* 23.)

"As regards the CONICAL CAPS worn by priests and the

mystery implied thereby it may be pointed out that the helmet of Pluto was the emblem of the generative principles hidden or undeveloped in the bosom of the earth."
—(Rolle, *Religions de la Grèce*, i., 68.)

"In studying the meaning of the FISH as an emblem sacred to Ishtar and Venus, we first notice its extraordinary fecundity. We next note that the fish selected is one which, when looked at from above, is almond-shaped. A gold carp may stand as the type of the sacred fish. To the surgeon or anatomist, to whom every part of the body is familiar, the side view of a carp is suggestive; the fork in the tail reminds him of what he knows as *la fourchette*. The accoucheur will remember how frequently he has heard of the *os tincæ*, and may recollect how anxious he was to catch a tench, that he might see the reason why the opening into the womb was called the tench's mouth. . . . . Putting these things together, we conclude that the fish was sacred because the form of its body represents one door, and the form of its mouth the other door, through which all the animal creation passes into life. The figure of a priest is given in one of the works on Nineveh, where part of the clothing consists of a big fish. The head of the minister is surmounted by its head, which, having its mouth open, indicates the origin of the BISHOP'S MITRE. As it would, of course, be inconvenient to wear the whole animal, the head was used to typify the body generally, and the mitre was formed to represent the head."—(Inman, *Ancient Faiths*, i., 111-112, 166.)

"The shape of the POMEGRANATE resembles that of the gravid uterus in the female, and the abundance of seeds which it contains makes it a fitting emblem of the prolific womb of the celestial mother. Its use was adopted largely in various forms of worship. In one part of Syria it was deified, and a temple erected in its honour."—(Inman, *Ancient Faiths*, ii., 611—12.

The LOTUS was the most sacred plant of the ancients, and typified the two principles of the earth's fecundation combined, the germ standing for the *Lingam*, the filaments and petals for the *Toni*. "Nympha signifies a young nubile woman, a certain part of the yoni and the calyx of roses; the lotus is a nymphæa. Hence a maiden is symbolised as being and having a ROSE, and the lotus typifies Isis and Sacti."—(Inman, *Ancient Faiths*, ii., 396.)

"The FIG-TREE is repeatedly joined with the vine by the sacred writers. Its Hebrew name is *tenah*, derived from a root which signifies 'to be crookened or bent;' also 'to copulate.' The word expressive of the fig-tree is the same as that used for *coitus.* It was of the leaves of this tree that aprons were made to cover our naked parents, and none can see the leaf without understanding the reason of the selection; it resembles the *trefoil*, the *fleur-de-lys*, and sundry other emblems suggestive of the triad. . . . . The fruit of the tree resembles in shape the virgin uterus. Its form led to the idea that it would promote fertility. To this day, in Oriental countries, the hidden meaning of the fig is almost as well known as its commercial value. . . . . We cannot doubt, when we put these considerations together, that 'to sit under the vine and fig-tree' was an expression equivalent to enjoying all the luxuries of life, as an old prayer-book expresses it, 'at bed and at board.' "— (Inman, *Ancient Faiths*, i., 526—8.)

"When speaking of the so-called Assyrian grove, I stated that the pine cone offered by priests to the deity, represented by that emblem, was typical of the " testes," the analogue of the mundane egg. In an ancient gem depicted by Maffei we notice the peculiar shape of the altar, the triple pillar arising from it, the ass's head and fictile offerings, the lad offering a pine cone surrounded with leaves, and carrying on his head a basket, in which two phalli are distinctly to be recognised. The deity to whom the sacrifice is offered is Bacchus, as figured by the people of Lampsacus. On his shoulder he bears a thyrsus, a wand or virga terminating in a pine cone, and having two ribbons dangling from it. We see, then, that amongst certain of the ancients the PINE CONE, the BASKET, and the THYRSUS were associated with Bacchus, or the solar deity under the male emblem. Out of twenty-seven gems figured by Raponi, in which the thyrsus occurs, in all it either indicates Bacchus or else is associated with such surrounding circumstances as to suggest an idea of licentious enjoyment. It is one of the emblems introduced into a representation of a female offering sacrifice to the god of Lampsacus. In two pictures, where the actors are drunk, the thyrsus has fallen down *abattu.* In Bacchic scenes the thyrsus is occasionally associated with the RING, the emblem of the female, and in one very significant scene, wherein Bacchus and Ariadne are seated upon a lioness, the pine cone and fillet are being caressed by the female."—(Inman, *Ancient Faiths*, ii., 490—493.)

" Mandrakes are like our plant the *Orchis mascula*, and their roots closely resemble the *scrotum* or the two testicles; consequently they were supposed to have potency in love affairs and were offered to Venus. There is a picture at Pompeii, in which a loving couple are presenting offerings

to the God of the Gardens, and amongst them the MAN-
DRAKE may be recognised. . . . . They are chiefly
interesting to us as an illustration of the close attention
paid by the ancients to those edibles which had, or were
supposed to have, an influence upon the organs which are
concerned in the creation of a new being. *Dudaim* are
only twice mentioned in the Bible (Genesis xxx. 14, 16,
and Song of Solomon vii. 13), and in both instances they
are connected with scenes of love. We may indeed consider that their name is derived from *dud*, 'love, that
which unites together.' I find from Royle that the
'atropa mandragora' is generally identified with love
apples. He says :—' The root is generally forked, and
closely resembles the lower part of the body of a man,
including the legs. The fruit is about the size of an
apple, very ruddy, of an agreeable odour, and is still
often eaten as exhilarating to the spirits and provocative
to venery . . . . . Reuben finds mandrakes and brings
them to Leah, the neglected wife of Jacob. With the
tempting fruit the patriarch becomes exhilarated, and, as
we conclude, unusually tender to his ugly spouse. Under
the influence of the charm we must also imagine that
the husband was prodigal in payment of the duties of
marriage, and to such a degree that the delighted wife
named the son who resulted from the union Issachar, not
because she had received her hire, *sachar*, but because
"she had had her fill," *shacar*. So far as we can learn there
was, in ancient times, an idea that any plant or animal
whose colour, appearance, and sometimes even whose
name, resembled that of any part of the body, was sure to
be useful in affections of that part. The *Orchis mascula*, whose roots are very remarkable for their shape,

was used whenever there was maleficia or impotentia, and the mandrake was employed for a similar purpose."— (*Ancient Faiths*, i., 338, ii., 250-251).

"According to the 'Doctrine of Signatures,' that the appearance of an object indicates the malady for which Nature has designed it for a remedy, the locust was employed as a medicine for certain affections of the genitals. A singular amulet illustrating this is figured by Caylus, a locust of the natural size, cut in agate, engraved on the base with the explanatory address to its influence, 'Locusta serva penem Tisicratis.' To explain the selection of this insect for such a purpose, it must be mentioned that the Greeks saw in its cylindrical, cambered, annulated body an analogy to the phallus; and hence its virtue as a *fascinum*, as its figure implied what the latter form actually represented. Hence Ecclesiastes' simile, 'the GRASSHOPPER shall be a burden,' alluding to the loss of virile power consequent on old age."—(King, *The Gnostics and their Remains*, 212-213.)

"The GOAT, on account of its genital member, was amongst the Egyptians placed in the ranks of the gods, for the same reason that the Greeks paid divine honours to Priapus. . . . . This animal being strongly inclined to the act of Venus, it was held that the member of his body which is the instrument of generation merited to be adored, because it is by this that Nature gives birth to all beings."—(*Diodorus Siculus*, lib. i., sec. 88.)

Dulaure says that the Greeks adored, under the names of Pan, Fauns, Satyrs, &c., rural deities whose figures at the same time represented the shape of the goat and the characteristic attribute of Priapus. They had the horns, sometimes the ears, and always the thighs, legs, and feet of the animal, and also the phallus in a state of vigour. "Temples have been raised to them; they are represented in a state of energy, *arrectis ita membra ut hirci naturam imitentui.*"—(*Diodorus Sic.,* lib. i., sec. 2.)

The FLAGELLUM in the hands of Osiris had its meaning, it being long known that flagellation served as a means for the restoration of virile power. According to Dr. Inman the crook, usually borne in his other hand, had also a connective hidden meaning difficult to indicate. He further traces a curious relation between the scourge and animals whose hides are marked with spots, and in connexion with whom it is frequently depicted. General Forlong points out, too, that Khem, an Egyptian phallic deity, is also furnished with a whip, "the quickener or exciter." Quoting from Mr. M'Clatchey's *China Revealed,* that "the old phallic gods, represented under two evident symbols, the Kheen or Yang, which is the *membrum virile,* and the Khw-an or Yin, the *pudendum muliebre,* or Yoni," he adds that "Yang, the agitator or whip, is seen acting on Yin, as representing receptive female *vis inertiæ.*"

Porphyrus says that the BULL chosen to fill the part of a god at Heliopolis had genital organs of extraordinary size, the better to denote the generative power that the sun exercises upon nature by its heat. Ammianus Marcellinus also says that the bull adored at Memphis had evident tokens of generative faculty.

Dulaure, in speaking of the most remarkable isolated phallus which Vivant Denon found at Thebes, in Upper Egypt, in a woman's tomb, says that this phallus (which had been a living organ) was embalmed and wrapped in bandages, and was found placed on the corresponding organ of

T

the female mummy. The engraving he gives of the mummy and the phallus proves that the latter was of more than natural size, and did not belong to the human species. "I am inclined to believe," he adds, "that the mummy was that of a woman of rank, and the embalmed phallus that of one of the sacred bulls, extracted after the animal's death, and placed in the tomb as a preservative against the evil spirits which the ancients believed tormented the souls of the dead. The Greeks and Romans sometimes placed figures of the phallus in sepulchres from a similar motive."—(Dulaure, *Histoire Abrégée des Cultes*, &c., ii., 56-57.)

Another animal was similarly honoured. "There is a place in Egypt called Chusea. The Aphrodite is worshipped in it, under the name of Urania. The people also worship a cow, and state, as a reason for their faith, that the cow belongs to this divinity. For the cow has an intense burning for copulation, and longs for it more than the male, so that when she hears the bellowing of the bull she becomes exceedingly excited and inflamed. . . . . The Isis herself, however, the Egyptians depict with horns like a cow."—(Ælian, *De Natur. Animal.*, x. 27.)

THE SYMBOL OF THE SERPENT.

" For a long period I was unable to see any significance in the adoption of the serpent as an emblem ; nor did I recognise it until I conversed with a gentleman who was familiar with the cobra in India. He told me that this snake and the Egyptian cerastes are both able to inflate the skin around the head, and to make themselves large and erect. In this they resemble the characteristic part of man ; consequently the serpent became a covert name and a mystic emblem. To this conclusion any one will readily assent who knows that in France the eel is used as a word embodying the same idea. . . . . When once we recognise the real signification of the symbol, we readily understand how it is that the serpent inserting a tail into a mouth symbolises eternity. A man perishes, yet man persists; the genus continues, through the constant reproduction of new scions from older branches. Yet there are no branches from the old stock, except by the union of father and mother. The symbol of union, therefore, becomes the sign of eternity, or rather of perpetuity; in other words, the emblem which we all regard without a qualm is nothing more than the mystic Adam and Eve, the 'zachar' (digger) and the 'nekebah' (hole), 'la queue et l'abricot fendu.' "—(Inman, *Ancient Faiths embodied in Ancient Names*, ii., 710, 712.)

"The connexion between life and that which is typified by the serpent is seen more conspicuously in the French language than in any other modern tongue which I am acquainted with. In it the phallus and existence have the same sound, the former [*le vit*] being, however, masculine, while the latter [*la vie*] is feminine" (*Ibid.*, i., 497-498). The same author describes a gem belonging to M. Lajard as follows : " The real age of the gem and its origin are not known, but the subject leads that author to believe it to be of late Babylonian workmanship. The stone is a white agate, shaped like a cone, and the cutting is on its lower face. The shape of this gem indicates its dedication to Venus. The central figure represents the androgyne deity Baalnu, Astaroth, Elohim, Jupiter genetrix, or the bearded Venus Mylitta. On the left side of the cutting we notice an erect serpent, whose rayed head makes us recognise the solar emblem and its mundane representative, *mentula arrecta ;* on a spot opposite to the centre of the male's body we find a lozenge symbolical of the yoni, whilst opposite to his feet is the amphora, whose mystic signification may readily be recognised—it is meant for Ouranos, or the Sun, fructifying Terra, or the Earth, by pouring from himself into her. The three stars over the head of the figure, and the inverted triangle on its head, are representations of the mythological four, equivalent to the Egyptian symbol of life. Opposite are the moon and another serpent of smaller size than that characterising the male, which may be readily recognised by physiologists as symbolic of *tensio clitoridis.* In a part corresponding to the diamond on the left side is a six-rayed wheel, emblematic, apparently, of the sun. At the female's feet is placed a cup, which is intended to represent the passive element in creation" (*Ibid.*, i., p. xiii.) Following the track of Dr. Donaldson, who in the Book of Jashar demonstrates that the word "akab," translated heel in Genesis xiii. 22, is a euphemism for *pudenda muliebria,* he holds that the interpretation of the sentence, "Thou shalt bruise his head, and he shall bruise thy heel," should be "Gloriam fascini congressio tollit et caput ejus humile facit, sed infligit injuriam moritura mentula quam impregnationem efficit et uteri per novas menses tumorem profert."—(*Ibid.*, i., 602.)

"We may rather ascribe the introduction of ophiolatry into Christian sects as the movement of a very considerable and intellectual body which rose into great importance in the second and third centuries, and which became prominent as a branch of the Nicolaitans and Gnostics. These affirmed (and truly, though they saw it not) that from the beginning God—that is, the Creator—had, in ophite form, manifested himself to the world, that 'he himself was of Draconic form,' and was that Serpent of Paradise which had on that occasion imparted wisdom and knowledge to our first parents (were they far wrong?); so these Christians kept serpents in baskets, chests, and arks, and their Eucharistic service consisted in opening an ark and enticing the serpent to come out by bits of bread, which having done, and folded himself about the bread, then he was a veritable Beth-el and Beth-lehem, and 'the sacrifice was complete;' the pious might then kiss the serpent, and the service was concluded by singing hymns to Almighty God. Such was but the continuance of services which had been very old when these began. Bacchanals well understood the consecrated cup and hymns to the Agatho-demon, and Demosthenes suffered severely for his eloquent denunciation against Æschines for being the bearer of such Bacchic and serpent mysteries. Delphi strictly kept its Sabbaths, or seven days, by similar hymns and mysteries to Python. A stranger at the Christian sacrament might see in its bits of bread a similar idea—the enticing of the Spirit."

"It would seem that the Caduceus of Mercury, that Rod of Life, is due to the fact of the ancients having observed that serpents conjoin in this double circular but erect form, as in Æsculapius' rod. Dr. C. E. Balfour, when at Ahmednagar in 1841, saw two living snakes drop into his garden, off the thatch of his bungalow, in a perfectly clear moonlight night. They were (he says) cobras, and stood erect as in the form of the Æsculapian rod, and no one could have seen them without at once recognising that they were in congress. It is a most fortunate thing, say Easterns, to see this, and if a cloth be then thrown over them, it becomes a form of Lakshmi, and of the highest procreative energy."—(Forlong, *Rivers of Life*, i., 223.)

THE RATIONALE OF GENERATION. — THE SACRIFICE OF VIRGINITY.—CONSECRATED WOMEN.—BRIDAL DEVOTIONS.

The Romans were accustomed to invoke the assistance of several deities in the matter of generation. Meursius (*Antiquities*, vol. v., De Puerperio) mentions Saturnus ut semen conferrit, Liber et Libera ut semen emitterent hic viris, illa feminis, Janus ut semeni in matricem commeanti januam aperiet, Juno et Mena ut flores menstruos regerent ad foetus concepti incrementum, Vitunus ut vitam daret, Sentinus ut sensum. St. Augustine (*De Civitate Dei*, lib. vi., cap. 9) completes the catalogue, adding, amongst others, Jugatinus, who brings the spouses together; Virginiea, who loosens the virginal zone; Volupia, who awakens desire; Stimula, who stimulates the husband; Strenia, who lends him the strength of which he has need; and does not forget Liber, who gives to the man invoking him a reproductive emission; whilst Libera accords the same favour, as it was then regarded, though ideas have somewhat changed on this point, to woman.

The young Hindus, according to Mendez Pinto, could not be received in Paradise with their virginity. Duquesne, in the neighbourhood of Pondicherry, saw brides make a complete sacrifice of their virginity to a wooden idol; and a similar custom obtained in the neighbourhood of Yra, where young girls offered the first fruits of Hymen to a similar idol with a Linga of iron, with which the sacrifice was effected. The custom also prevailed amongst the ancients. At Biblos young girls had the alternative of prostituting themselves for a whole day to strangers or of sacrificing their hair to the goddess. If we may judge by the lively outcries raised by different writers against this worship of the Venus of Biblos, and against its indecency, it is evident that the girls of this city preferred to " keep their hair on."

In ancient Palestine generally, and even in Jerusalem itself, we find two distinct words are used to indicate prostitution; the first, " kadesh," signifies " a consecrated one ;" the second is " zanah," whose primary meaning is *semen emittere.* The distinction between the two is very much the same as that which obtains between the "bebis" of India and the temple women, the " zanahs" being those who adopt the practice from love of lucre or from passion, whilst the " kedeshah" adopted it mainly from a religious feeling. When the law was enunciated that the hire of a whore and the price of a dog should not be brought into the house of the Lord for any vow, the words used are *zanah* and *celeb,* so that we do not take it to apply to the consecrated ones. . . . . The kedeshim seem to have worn a peculiar dress, by which they could be recognised. When Tamar wished to entice Judah, she arrayed herself like a consecrated one, and the patriarch thought her a *Kedeshah,* and conse-quently one with whom he might legitimately go.— (Inman, *Ancient Faiths,* ii., 175—177.)

Amongst the Romans Mutinus, or Tutinus, seems to have been the name given to the isolated PHALLUS, and PRIAPUS to that attached to a Hermes or other figure. Under either form it was held to preside over the fertility

of women and the sources of conjugal vigour. In consequence of these supposed virtues brides, before being
delivered over to their husbands' embraces, were conducted by their parents to one of these images, and, with
heads covered by a veil, seated themselves on the most
salient portion. St. Augustine says on this subject, "A
custom thought to be very proper and very religious
amongst the Roman ladies is that of obliging brides to
seat themselves upon the monstrous and superabundant
fascinum of a Priapus" (*De Civitate Dei*, vi., 9). So
Lactantius would seem to refer to the practice obtaining
in some Oriental countries of the sacrifice being entirely
accomplished by the god of wood or iron in the passage. "And Mutinus, on whose extremity brides seat
themselves in order that the god may appear to have received the first sacrifice of their modesty" (*De Falsâ Reli-
gione*). Possibly the jealousy of the Roman bridegrooms
put a limit to such complete devotion, though a certain
contact was, no doubt, deemed needful to render the
ceremony complete, assure fecundity, and neutralise spells
and enchantments directed against a happy consummation
of the union. Married women also followed this practice
in order to destroy the charm that rendered them sterile,
but, more hardened than the brides, they carried their
devotion further. "Do not you yourselves lead your
wives to Tutinus, and, to destroy alleged enchantments,
do not you make them bestride the immense and horrible
fascinum?" (*Arnobius*, lib. 4.) A group engraved by
Meursius from the gallery at Florence gives a representation of this ceremony. A woman, with her head
covered by a kind of cap, stands with her hands engaged
in supporting her uplifted garments, leaving a part of her

body exposed. An enormous Phallus rears itself from the ground as far as the sexual organs of the figure. These, which are visibly proportioned on a large scale, seem to be in contact with the upper end of the Phallus. The custom is, indeed, far from obsolete. "Many a day," says General Forlong, "have I stood at early dawn at the door of my tent, pitched in a sacred grove, and gazed at the little groups of females stealthily emerging from the adjoining half-sleeping village, each with a little garland or bunch of sweet flowers, and perhaps costly oil, wending their way to that temple in the grove or garden of the god and goddess of creation, and when none were thought to see, accompanying their earnest prayer for Pooli-Palam (child-fruit) with a respectful abrasion of a certain part of their person on Linga-jee and a little application of the drippings that are for ever trickling from the orifice of the Argha" (Forlong, *Rivers of Life*, i., 205). So Dr. Inman, speaking of the upright and circular stone so common in Oriental villages, says, "The two indicate the male and female, and a medical friend resident in India has told me that he has seen women mount upon the lower stone and seat themselves reverently upon the upright-one, having first adjusted their dress so as to prevent it interfering with their perfect contact with the miniature obelisc. During the sitting a short prayer seemed flitting over the worshipper's lips, but the whole affair was soon over."

"When speaking of the so-called Assyrian grove I stated that the pine cone offered by priests to the deity represented by that emblem was typical of the testis, the analogue of the mundane egg. In an ancient gem depicted by Maffei we notice the peculiar shape of the altar, the triple pillar arising from it, the ass's head and fictile offerings, the lad offering a pine cone surrounded with leaves, and carrying on his head a basket in which two phalli are distinctly to be recognised. The deity to whom the sacrifice is offered is Bacchus, as figured by the people of Lampsacus. On his shoulder he bears a thyrsus, a wand or virga, terminating in a pine cone, and having two ribbons dangling from it. We see, then, that amongst certain of the ancients, the ASS, the PINE CONE, the BASKET, and the THYRSUS were associated with Bacchus, or the solar deity under the male emblem. Out of twenty-seven gems figured by Raponi, in which the thyrsus occurs, in all it either indicates Bacchus, or else is associated with such surrounding circumstances as to suggest an idea of licentious enjoyment. It is one of the emblems introduced into a representation of a female, offering sacrifice to the god of Lampsacus. In two pictures, where the actors are drunk, the thyrsus has fallen down *abattu.* In Bacchic scenes the thyrsus is occasionally associated with the RING, the emblem of the female; and in one very significant scene, wherein Bacchus and Ariadne are seated upon a lioness, the pine cone and fillet are being caressed by the female."—(Inman, *Ancient Faiths*, ii., 490—493.)

THE RELIGIOUS RITES OF ANCIENT ROME.

General Forlong, in his "Rivers of Life," has dealt at great length with the essentially phallic basis underlying the religion of Rome, but hitherto all but ignored by writers on what is usually styled classic mythology. He identifies the Palatine Hill as that dedicated from the earliest times to the male energy, and the Capitoline as that sacred especially to the female cult, to which he holds the Romans were, as a rule, more addicted. He further traces the erection of Lignean phallic gods, afterwards succeeded by Fire and Solar deities, in various parts of the city. Of the survivals of purely phallic worship evidence abounds, and also of the fact that women were generally the more active participants. St. Augustine says :—"The sexual member of man is consecrated in the temple of Liber, that of woman in the sanctuaries of Libera, the same goddess as Venus, and these two divinities are called the father and the mother because they preside over the act of generation" (*De Civitate Dei*, vi., 9). Liber was a title of Bacchus, in whose honour the festival of the Liberales was held in March, six days after the Greeks celebrated their Dionysia, in honour of the same divinity. The Phallus, styled by the Romans Mutinus or Tutinus, when isolated from the representation of a human figure, played a prominent part in these celebrations. On the authority of Varro, St. Augustine states that at certain places in Italy this emblem, placed upon a chariot, was solemnly and with great honour drawn about the fields, the highways, and finally the towns. "At Lavinium the festival of the god Liber lasted a month, during which all gave themselves up to pleasure, licentiousness and debauchery. Lascivious ditties and the freest speech were kept company by like actions. A magnificent car bearing an enormous Phallus was slowly drawn to the centre of the forum, where it came to a halt, and the most respectable matron of the town advanced and crowned this obscene image with a wreath" (*De Civitate Dei*, vii., 21). Some days later was celebrated the festival of Venus, also associated at Rome with the emblem of virility. During this festival the

Roman ladies proceeded in state to the Quirinal, where stood the temple of the Phallus, took possession of this sacred object, and escorted it in procession to the temple of Venus Erycina, where they placed it in the bosom of the goddess. A cornelian gem,* with a representation of this ceremony upon it, has been engraved in the "Culte Secret des Dames Romaines." A triumphal chariot bears a kind of altar, on which rests a colossal Phallus. A genius hovering above this object holds a crown of flowers suspended over it. The chariot and genius are under a square canopy, supported at the four corners by spears, each borne by a semi-nude woman. The chariot is drawn by goats and bulls, ridden by winged children, and is preceded by a group of women blowing trumpets. Further on, and in front of the car, is an object characteristic of the female sex, representing the *sinus veneris.* This emblem, the proportions of which correspond to those of the Phallus on the chariot, is upheld by two genii. These appear to be pointing out to the Phallus the place it is to occupy. The ceremony accomplished, the Roman ladies devoutly escorted the Phallus back to its temple. The mysteries of Bacchus were celebrated at Rome in the temple of that god and in the sacred wood near the Tiber, styled Simila. At the outset women alone were admitted to these ceremonies, which took place in the daytime. A woman of Campania, named Pacculla Minia, on being made priestess, entirely changed the nature of the institution by initiating her two sons, and decreeing that the mysteries should only be celebrated by night. Other men were introduced, and with them

---

* See page 108, "Fig. XXV." A copy of this gem will be given among our illustrations.

frightful disorders. The youths admitted were never more than twenty years of age. Introduced by the priests into subterranean vaults, the young initiate was exposed to their brutality, whilst frightful yells and the din of drums and cymbals served to drown the outcries their violence might provoke. Wine flowing in abundance stimulated excesses, which the shade of night further favoured. Age and sex were confounded, all shame was cast aside, and every species of luxury, even that contrary to nature, sullied the temple of the divinity. If any of the young initiates resisted the importunities of the libertine priests and priestesses, and acquitted themselves negligently in the peculiar duties expected from them, they were sacrificed by being attached to machines, which suddenly plunged them into lower caverns, where they met their death. The priests accounted for their disappearance by ascribing it to the action of the god whom they were alleged to have offended. Shouting and dancing by men and women, supposed to be moved by divine influence, formed a leading episode in these ceremonies. Women with dishevelled hair were seen to plunge lighted torches, chemically prepared beforehand, into the waters of the Tiber without extinguishing them. At these midnight assemblies poisons were brewed, wills forged, perjuries arranged, and murders planned. The initiates were of all classes, even the very highest, and their numbers became so great that they were regarded as a danger to the State, against which they are said to have plotted. Consequently the Senate, on the representations of the Consul Posthumius, abolished these assemblies A.U.C. 564. Juvenal, in his Sixth Satire, has spoken in terms hardly quotable of the excesses practised at the festival of the Bona Dea.

General Forlong has also a few general observations upon the marked Phallo-Fire worship of the Greeks and Romans, too commonly called 'Fire and Ancestor Worship.' The signs or Nishāns of the generating parents—that is, the Lares and Penates—were placed in the family niches close to the holy flame—that "hot air," "holy spirit," or "breath," the active force of the Hebrew B R A, and the Egyptian P'ta, the "engenderer of the heavens and earth," before which ignorant and superstitious races prayed and prostrated themselves, just as they do to-day before very similar symbols. The Greeks and Romans watched over their fires as closely as do our Parsees or Zoroastrians. The males of the family had to see that the holy flame never went out, but in the absence of the head of the house, and practically at all times, this sacred duty devolved on the matron of the house. Every evening the sacred fire was carefully covered with ashes, so that it might not go out by oversight, but quietly smoulder on ; and in the morning the ashes were removed, when it was brightened up and worshipped. In March, or early spring, it was allowed to die out, but not before the New Year's Fire had been kindled from Sol's rays and placed in the Sanctuary. No unclean object was allowed to come near Agni; none durst ever warm themselves near him ; nor could any blameworthy action take place in his presence. He was only approached for adoration or prayer ; not as Fire, which he was not, but as sexual flame, or Life. . . . . It seems extraordinary to Asiatics, as I have often found when conversing with them about Roman faiths, and what Europeans believe in regard to these, that this matter is still so misunderstood in Europe, where the worship of the Lares and Penates is usually held to be in some mysterious way the worship of the dead and the ancestors of the household. No clear attempt has yet been made to unravel this subject from the confusion in which it lies, and to set forth in their true light those gods. The real pith of the matter is briefly this, that Penates are Lingams, or male organs; and Lares, Yonis, or female organs. These symbols often doubtless represented ancestry, but rather grossly so, before the days of statuary and painting, and were placed over the family hearth just as we still place there the pictures or forms of our great dead ones. So in family niches near the sacred fire we see, as I have often done in secret nooks of Indian domiciles, small rudely-formed figures in stone or baked clay, elongated when these were Penates and represented males, but ovate when Lares, or the female dead of the tribe or family. . . . . As the cremated dead, and those whose bodies bleached on a foreign shore, had no tombstones, it was necessary, in order to have them in remembrance, to place some fitting symbol or relic of them near the god of the household, the sacred fire. This was not Phallic worship exactly, yet Lares and Penates are Phalli. The Lares and Penates represented the past vital fire or energy of the tribe, as the patriarch, his stalwart sons and daughters, did that of the present living fire on the sacred hearth.—(Forlong, *Rivers of Life*, i., 387—389.)

SACRED COLOURS—BELLS IN ANCIENT WORSHIP—THE
COCK AS AN EMBLEM.

Dr. Inman notes that there is something mystical about red as a colour, though the philologist will readily understand why it should be adopted by the followers of

Mahadevi. Rams' skins dyed red were ordered for the Jewish tabernacle (Exodus xxv. 5). Scarlet, cedar-wood, and hyssop were burnt with the red heifer used in the water of separation (Numbers xix. 6). In the Romish Church the highest dignitaries wear scarlet and purple. Red powder is used in Hindu worship, Jaganath is painted red, and for a priest to throw the powder on a woman's breast is equivalent to soliciting adultery. Colonel Forbes Leslie notes that what he styles the "excluded member" of an Indian stone circle, the situation of which he likens to that of the Friar's Heel at Stonehenge, was daubed with white patches, with a red mark in the centre, and recalls the vermilion oil and minium used to smear Jove's statue or symbol at Rome on festal days. "This is still the practice all over India, showing how closely Greece and Rome have followed the Indian cult. Especially is it used for Omphi, or rotund egg-like objects, a protruding ovate face of a tree or rock; under such a tree there would sure to be seen or imagined, and immediately depicted, an Eva, Chavah, or cleft. The nature of this besmearing shows the object is dedicated to the deities of fertility, red oil and water meaning this all over the East, for obvious reasons. . . . . I have often availed myself of a religious feeling by marking lines if running over rocks or stones or on trees with red-coloured lines or dots, red being Parvati's hue, fertility, and much as the cultivator feared to see a theodolite levelled across his family soil, he would never try to efface the red marks unless he was an educated sceptic, which our schools and chief cities have not been slow to produce, and which we thankfully welcome."—(Forlong, *Rivers of Life.*)

"Priapus was represented with the head of Pan or

the Fauns—that is to say, with goat's horns and ears.
When he had arms—for he was not always found with
them—Priapus held in one hand a scythe, and sometimes
with his left hand grasped, like Osiris, the characteristic
feature of his divinity, which was always colossal, threaten-
ing, and painted red. . . . . All the figures of Priapus
were not thus coarsely made; some were wrought with
care, as well as the Termi forming the lower part. That
which the figure bore here was stark naked and painted
red."—(Dulaure, *Histoire Abrégée de différens Cultes*, ii.,
169-170.)

"No Lingam worship can be conducted without the
bell; in union the Lingam and bell give forth life and
sound, as Siva's priests have confessed to me. Bell
ornamentation is very conspicuous on sacred buildings,
where it is usually said to represent the mammæ, and
denote fertility. A copper vase found at Cairo shows
us Isis as the nursing mother, forming, together with her
boy, a 'Column of Life,' inside what we may call 'the
Assyrian Tree or Door of Life,' or the Jewish 'Grove.'
The bell flowers around them are held to be the Ciborium
or Egyptian bean, and to represent both a bell and a teat,
whilst the matured bean was thought very like the
male organ. . . . . Near the furthest western source of
the Tay, amongst the most rugged and lofty scenery of
Perthshire, lies the Scottish 'Pool of Bethesda,' here called
the Holy Pool of Strathfillan, a centre for unknown ages
of healing efficacy, of blessing and superstition. Near to
this pool, site of the old Druidic shrine of Felan, Balan,
or Faolan, did the new faith erect its ancient church of
St. Fillan, and appropriated the old Sivaik bell of conical
shape and phallic handle. Truly, as the Lord Bishop of

Brechin says in his account of this bell, 'the handle is the most remarkable part, for there we find twice repeated the well-known heathen emblem of the phallus.' "— (Forlong, *Rivers of Life*, i., 232-233 ; ii., 299-300.)

The passage, "Moreover, because the daughters of Zion are haughty . . . . walking and mincing as they go, and making a tinkling with their feet" (Isaiah iii. 16), implies that they too wore bells as an ornament. "No greater reproach can be cast upon a woman than that she has carried into married life the evidence of precedent impurity. Those who are familiar with the Mosaic law will remember the stress laid upon 'the tokens of virginity,' and the importance which the mother attached to being able to produce them for her daughter. There is a belief that what physiologists call 'the hymen' may be destroyed by such an accident as too long a stride in walking, running, or stepping over a stile, or by a single jump. To prevent the possibility of such an occurrence, and the casualty which it involves, all maidens have their dress furnished with a light cord or chain about the level of the knees. This enables them to take short paces, but not to 'straddle' over anything. To make the fetter as ornamental as possible, the ligature is furnished with bells. This custom is referred to in the sentence above quoted. The custom also prevailed in ancient Arabia, as is evident from Mohammed's injunction in the Koran, 'Let them (the women) not make a noise with their feet, that the ornaments they hide may not be discovered.' When marriage is consummated there is no occasion for the use of the jingling chain. 'To bear away the bell,' therefore, is equivalent to 'taking a virgin to wife.' In Pompeii and Herculaneum, where paintings still tell us of the inner

life of Italian and Grecian cities, a vast number of bronzes
and pictures have been found, in which the phallus is
adorned with one or more bells. The intention is clearly
to show that, like Solomon, it had many wives, all of
whom brought with them the tokens of virginity."—
(Inman, *Ancient Faiths*, i., 53-54.)

"Gall, or Gallus, is a cock and a swan, both emblems of
the Sun and Jove. That there is a bond of union apparently between Gallus and Phallus is often forced upon
our notice, as in the figure given by Payne Knight, where
the body of a man has for its head the figure of a cock,
of which the beak is the phallus, whilst on the pediment
below is written ' *Soter Kosmou*, Saviour of the World,' a
term applied to all gods, but especially those charged with
creative functions. Minerva, who is also called Pallas,
is very often shown with a cock sitting on her helmet,
and her crest denotes her *penchant* for this salacious
bird. . . . . I have mentioned the sacrifice of the cock
by Celts; it was and still is over all Asia the cheap,
common and very venial substitute for man. The princes
of India can afford the *Aswa-meda* or great horse sacrifice,
and a Syrian Patriarch, a ram ' caught in the thicket,'
and burn it instead of his child, on the mountain altar, to
his mountain Jahveh; but it is more common now to see
the morning announcer of the ' Sun of Righteousness,'
the impetuous king of the village middens, being quietly
conveyed up the mountain pass to die for his Lord, instead
of a ram or child. Many a time have I followed the
sacrificing party up some sacred defile to the summit god,
and watched the pitiful gaze of several poor followers who
saw their favourite and beautiful bird about to be sacrificed, by having its blood bespattered by cruel, priestly

hands over their 'Rock of Ages,' the Tsur-oo-Salem. The poor owners had never probably been asked, or if so in a way which brooked not refusal, if they would yield up to their deity the cheery announcer of their uneventful days of labour; for in general the selection falls on the finest bird of the village, and the actual sacrificers are rarely those who lose anything by the transaction. In this I speak of the customs of rude Indian tribes; but such sacrifices were also common to and performed in much the same way by Phœnicians, Scyths, Sueves, Jews, Greeks, &c. The horse was also sacrificed by all peoples at some period of their history; but the cock has been the enduring favourite, and cruelly though he has been treated, wherever a Sabean or phallic altar has been raised, his pre-eminence has been acknowledged. As an emblem of a world-wide idea he still divides the right to rule on the temples and spires of Christian Europe, and on the humbler shrines of many nations, with the Crescent of Isis and Arabia, and the Tau or Cross, that ancient "wood of health" (Forlong, *Rivers of Life*, i., 383; ii., 274-5). "The connexion between the cock, the sun, and the idea of masculinity, has existed from the earliest known times to the present. The union of ideas appears to be—1. That the cock proclaims the sunrise. 2. That the cock is for its size unusually strong, plucky, and courageous. 3. That it seems to have unlimited powers amongst the hens."—(Inman, *Ancient Faiths*, i., 536-537.)

INDEX.

THE END.

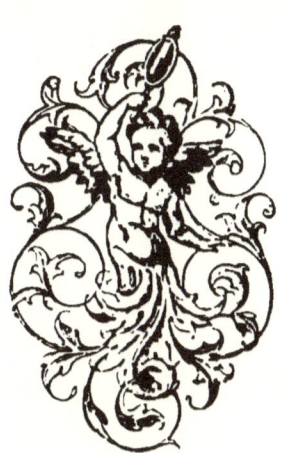

𝕸𝖗. 𝕽𝖊𝖉𝖜𝖆𝖞'𝖘 𝕻𝖚𝖇𝖑𝖎𝖈𝖆𝖙𝖎𝖔𝖓𝖘.

—◦✦◦—

In crown 8vo, in French grey wrapper, uniform with the Bibliographies of
Ruskin, Dickens, Thackeray, *and* Carlyle. *Price* 6s.
A few copies on Large Paper. Price 10s. 6d.

The Bibliography of Swinburne;

A Bibliographical List, arranged in Chronological Order, of the Published Writings in Verse and Prose

OF

ALGERNON CHARLES SWINBURNE
(1857-1884).

This Bibliography commences with the brief-lived College Magazine, to which Mr. Swinburne was one of the chief contributors when an undergraduate at Oxford in 1857-58. Besides a careful enumeration and description of the first editions of all his separately published volumes and pamphlets in verse and prose, the original appearance is duly noted of every poem, prose article, or letter, contributed to any journal or magazine (*e.g.,* Once-a-Week, *The Spectator,* The Cornhill Magazine, *The Morning Star, The Fortnightly Review, The Examiner, The Dark Blue, The Academy, The Athenæum, The Tatler, Belgravia, The Gentleman's Magazine, La République des Lettres, Le Rappel, The Glasgow University Magazine, The Daily Telegraph,* &c., &c.), whether collected or uncollected. Among other entries will be found a remarkable novel, published in instalments and never issued in a separate form, and several productions in verse not generally known to be from Mr. Swinburne's pen. The whole forms a copious and it is believed approximately complete record of a remarkable and brilliant literary career, extending already over a quarter of a century.

** *Only 250 copies printed.*

———

A "Rosicrucian" Book.
In demy 8vo, cloth. Price £1 1s.

Phallicism:

Celestial and Terrestrial, Heathen and Christian, its connection with the Rosicrucians and the Gnostics, and its foundation in Buddhism. With an Essay on Mystic Anatomy. By Hargrave Jennings, author of "The Rosicrucians."

In 12mo, cloth (Subscribers only).

Lord Byron and His Works.

A Biography and Essay. Translated from the Italian of CESARE CANTÙ. Edited, with Notes and Appendix, by A. KINLOCH. Dedicated (by permission) to his Excellency the MARQUIS OF LORNE, K.T.

. Among the Subscribers are the MARQUIS of RIPON, the MARQUIS of LORNE, the EARL of NORTHBROOK, F.M. LORD NAPIER of MAGDALA, and General Sir WM. F. WILLIAMS, Bart.

REDWAY'S SHILLING SERIES, VOL. III.

Édition de Luxe in demy 18mo.

Tobacco Talk and Smokers' Gossip.

An Amusing Miscellany of Fact and Anecdote relating to "The Great Plant" in all its Forms and Uses, including a Selection from Nicotian Literature.

In crown 8vo, cloth. Price 3s. 6d.

Sandracoltus; a Drama.

By W. THEODORE SMITH.

"A small but very wondrous book."—*Academy.*

In crown 8vo, cloth. Price 5s.

The Angelic Pilgrim,

An Epical History of the Chaldee Empire. By W. H. WATSON.

"An epical poem of considerable length and beauty . . . an historic narrative of the Chaldee Empire, its rise and fall, and the influence it exercised on the prehistoric world."—*Christian Union.*

In crown 8vo, 5s.; cloth, 6s.

A Study in Social Physiology.

Prostitution under the Regulation System. Translated from the French of M. YVES GUYOT by E. B. TRUMAN, M.D., F.C.S. With 25 Diagrams.

Bibliotheca Arcana, Seu Catalogus Librorum Penetralium,

Being Brief Notices of Books that have been Secretly Printed, Prohibited by Law, Seized, Anathematised, Burnt or Bowdlerised. [*Prospectus on application.*]

REPRINTED FROM THE UNIQUE ORIGINAL [BOSTON, 1827].

Tamerlane and Other Poems.

By EDGAR ALLAN POE. Edited, with an Introduction, by R. H. SHEP-HERD. Printed in the best style on Whatman paper at the Chiswick Press.

₊ *100 copies only. Price £1 1s.*

"A veritable *livre de luxe* . . . this will be held dear to the bibliophile, whilst to the world at large the work possesses especial interest as being that first published by EDGAR ALLAN POE, in Boston, in 1827; and the specimen copy from which this was printed is unique."—*Society.*

In crown 8vo, parchment. Price 2s. 6d.

The Anatomy of Tobacco;

OR SMOKING METHODISED, DIVIDED AND CONSIDERED AFTER A NEW FASHION.

By LEOLINUS SILURIENSIS.

In demy 8vo, with Illustrative Plates. Price 1s. 6d.

Chirognomancy;

OR INDICATIONS OF TEMPERAMENT AND APTITUDES MANI-FESTED BY THE FORM AND TEXTURE OF THE THUMB AND FINGERS.

By ROSA BAUGHAN.

"Miss Baughan has already established her fame as a writer upon occult subjects, and what she has to say is so very clear and so easily verified that it comes with the weight of authority."—*Lady's Pictorial.*

In post 4to, vellum. Price £1 1s.

The Divine Pymander

OF HERMES MERCURIUS TRISMEGISTUS.

IN XVII. BOOKS.

Translated from the Arabic by Dr. EVERARD, 1650. New Edition, edited with Introductory Essay by HARGRAVE JENNINGS, author of "The Rosicrucians."

₊ *Edition limited to 200 copies.*

Phallic Worship.

By HODDER M. WESTROPP. With Illustrations.   [*In preparation.*

Édition de luxe, in demy 18mo. *Price* 1s.

Confessions of an English Hachish Eater.

"There is a sort of bizarre attraction in this fantastic little book, with its weird, unhealthy imaginations."—*Whitehall Review.*

In crown 8vo, cloth. Price 4s. 6d.

Theosophy, Religion, and Occult Science,

COLLECTED ADDRESSES.

By COLONEL HENRY S. OLCOTT, President of the Theosophical Society.

THE ONLY PUBLISHED BIOGRAPHY OF JOHN LEECH.
An édition de luxe in demy 18mo. *Price* 1s.

John Leech, Artist and Humourist:

A Biographical Sketch. By FRED. G. KITTON. New Edition, revised.

"In the absence of a fuller biography we cordially welcome Mr. Kitton's interesting little sketch."—*Notes and Queries.*

"The multitudinous admirers of the famous artist will find this touching monograph well worth careful reading and preservation."—*Daily Chronicle.*

"The very model of what such a memoir should be."—*Graphic.*

THACKERAY AND CRUIKSHANK.

The only "verbatim" reprint of the most charming of THACKERAY'S critical Essays.

In demy 8vo, *wrappered, uniform with* "*Phiz*" *and* "*Leech.*" *Price* 3s. 6d. *A few large paper copies, with India proof portrait, in imperial* 8vo, *parchment. Price* 7s. 6d.

An Essay on the Genius of George Cruikshank,

By "Theta" (WILLIAM MAKEPEACE THACKERAY). With all the Original Woodcut Illustrations, a New Portrait of CRUIKSHANK, etched by PAILTHORPE, and a Prefatory Note on THACKERAY AS AN ART CRITIC, by W. E. CHURCH, Secretary of the Urban Club.

In demy 8vo, with Illustrative Plates. Price 1s.

The Handbook of Palmistry,

Including an Account of the Doctrines of the Kabbala. By R. BAUGHAN,
Author of " Indications of Character in Handwriting."

"It possesses a certain literary interest, for Miss Baughan shows the
connection between palmistry and the doctrines of the Kabbala."—*Graphic.*

"Miss Rosa Baughan, for many years known as one of the most expert
proficients in this branch of science, has as much claim to consideration as
any writer on the subject."—*Sussex Daily News.*

"People who wish to believe in Palmistry, or the science of reading
character from the marks of the hand," says the *Daily News*, in an article
devoted to the discussion of this topic, "will be interested in a handbook
of the subject by Miss Baughan, published by Mr. Redway."

---

*Printed on large (hand-made) paper, with India Proof Illustrations mounted
as Frontispiece and Tailpiece. Price £1 11s. 6d.*

The Worship of Priapus.

Being an Account of the Fête of ST. COSMO and DAMIANO, celebrated at
ISERNIA. In a letter to SIR JOSEPH BANKS, President of the Royal Society.
By SIR WILLIAM HAMILTON, Minister at the Court of Naples. To which is
added SOME ACCOUNT OF PHALLIC WORSHIP, principally derived from the
Work of RICHARD PAYNE KNIGHT. Edited, with Preface and Notes, by
HARGRAVE JENNINGS, author of "The Rosicrucians."

*** *Only 100 copies printed, each numbered.*

---

*In demy 8vo, elegantly printed on Dutch hand-made paper, and bound in
parchment-paper cover. Price 1s.*

The Scope and Charm of Antiquarian Study.

By JOHN BATTY, F.R.Hist.S., Member of the Yorkshire Archæological and
Topographical Association.

"It forms a useful and entertaining guide to a beginner in historical
researches."—*Notes and Queries.*

"The author has laid it before the public in a most inviting, intelligent,
and intelligible form, and offers every incentive to the study in every
department, including Ancient Records, Manorial Court-Rolls, Heraldry,
Painted Glass, Mural Paintings, Pottery, Church Bells, Numismatics, Folk-
Lore, &c., to each of which the attention of the student is directed. The
pamphlet is printed on a beautiful modern antique paper, appropriate to
the subject of the work."—*Brighton Examiner.*

"Mr. Batty, who is one of those folks Mr. Dobson styles 'gleaners
after time,' has clearly and concisely summed up, in the space of a few
pages, all the various objects which may legitimately be considered to
come within the scope of antiquarian study."—*Academy.*

EBENEZER JONES' POEMS.

In post 8vo, cloth, old style. Price 5s.

Studies of Sensation and Event.

Poems by EBENEZER JONES. Edited, Prefaced, and Annotated by RICHARD HERNE SHEPHERD. With Memorial Notices of the Author by SUMNER JONES and W. J. LINTON. A new Edition. With Photographic Portrait of the Poet.

"This remarkable poet affords nearly the most striking instance of neglected genius in our modern school of poetry. His poems are full of vivid disorderly power."—D. G. ROSSETTI.

In crown 8vo, with Engraved Frontispiece. Price 5s.

R. H. Horne's Cosmo de' Medici:

An Historical Tragedy, and other Poems. By RICHARD HENGIST HORNE, Author of "Orion." FOURTH EDITION.

"We have been among the earliest readers of Mr. Horne—among the most ardent admirers of his high genius—for a man of high, of the highest genius, he unquestionably is."—EDGAR ALLAN POE.

"I have been diving into his treasure house (COSMO DE' MEDICI) this morning, with keen delight and admiration."—ALGERNON CHARLES SWINBURNE.

"This tragedy is the work of a poet and not of a playwright. Many of the scenes abound in vigour and tragic intensity. If the structure of the drama challenges comparison with the masterpieces of the Elizabethan stage, it is at least not unworthy of the models which have inspired it."—*Times.*

Specimen Number sent Post Free for Two Shillings.

The Theosophist.

A Monthly Journal devoted to Oriental Philosophy, Art, Literature and Occultism; embracing Mesmerism, Spiritualism and other Secret Sciences. Conducted by H. P. BLAVATSKY.

THE THEOSOPHIST is issued monthly, and the subscription is £1 for twelve numbers of not less than 48 columns royal 4to of reading matter, or 576 columns in all, *including postage.*

With the issue of OCTOBER (1884) will commence the SIXTH VOLUME of this journal.

Theosophy has suddenly risen to importance . . . The movement implied by the term Theosophy is one that cannot be adequately explained in a few words . . . those interested in the movement, which is not to be confounded with spiritualism, will find means of gratifying their curiosity by procuring the back numbers of *The Theosophist* and a very remarkable book called *Isis Unveiled,* by Madame Blavatsky.—*Literary World.*

LONDON: GEORGE REDWAY, YORK STREET, COVENT GARDEN.

[Appointed Agent for the Theosophical Society's Publications.]

Mr. HARGRAVE JENNINGS' WORKS.